CRASH COURSE

Ethics and Human Sciences

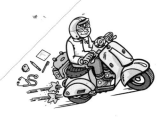

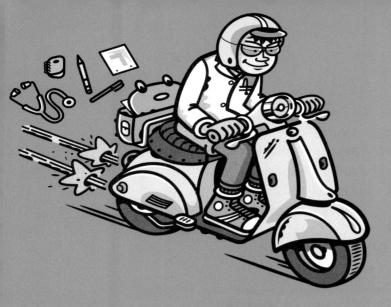

Series editor
Daniel Horton-Szar
BSc (Hons) MBBS (Hons)
Northgate Medical Practice
Canterbury

Faculty advisors
Sarah Edwards
BSc MA PhD
Senior Lecturer in Research Governance
Research and Development Directorate
University College London Hospitals NHS Trust

Richard W. Morris
PhD
Reader in Medical Statistics and Epidemiology
Department of Primary Care and Population
Sciences
Royal Free and University College Medical
School
University of London

Mike Porter
BA (Hons) MPhil
Senior Lecturer
Division of Community Health Sciences:
General Practice
University of Edinburgh

Ethics and
Human Sciences

Keith Amarakone
MBChB BSc (Hons) MA
Senior House Officer
Royal Cornwall Hospital
Truro

Sukhmeet S. Panesar
BSc (Hons)
Imperial College London
University of London

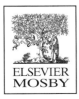

ELSEVIER
MOSBY

Edinburgh • London • New York • Oxford • Philadelphia • St Louis • Sydney • Toronto 2006

ELSEVIER
MOSBY

Commissioning Editor	**Fiona Conn**
Project Manager	**Frances Affleck**
Designer	**Andy Chapman**
Cover Illustration	**Kevin Faerber**
Illustration Manager	**Bruce Hogarth**
Illustrator	**PCA Creative**

First published 2006

ISBN (10): 0723433461
ISBN (13): 9780723433460

British Library Cataloguing in Publication Data
A catalogue record for this book is available from the British Library

Library of Congress Cataloging in Publication Data
A catalog record for this book is available from the Library of Congress

Notice
Neither the Publisher nor the Authors assume any responsibility for any loss or injury and/or damage to persons or property arising out of or related to any use of the material contained in this book. It is the responsibility of the treating practitioner, relying on independent expertise and knowledge of the patient, to determine the best treatment and method of application for the patient.

The Publisher

ELSEVIER your source for books, journals and multimedia in the health sciences
www.elsevierhealth.com

Printed in Italy

The publisher's policy is to use paper manufactured from sustainable forests

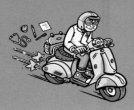

Preface

Medical ethics, sociology and epidemiology rarely arouse one's passion and can, as minor subjects within a busy curriculum, find themselves ignored by vast swathes of students. However, recent times have seen not only a greater general understanding of these subjects but also a greater appreciation of their role within modern medical practice.

In addition, these subjects are increasingly appearing in exams and, more importantly, they will crop up in every field and at every level of your working lives. In writing this book, we hope to provide a springboard from which you can develop a reasoned ethical approach to dilemmas as and when they present to you, both within your practice of medicine and in the exam situation. The sociology and public health sections aim to provide key information on the theories and studies that have helped to shape the practice of these disciplines – topics that are all too often unacknowledged by medical students and doctors alike. In doing so, we hope to provide you with the essential facts on these subjects without leaving you to wade through irrelevant material. Hopefully, all students might begin to enjoy evidence (as well as experience)-based medicine and appreciate its importance regardless of the medical or surgical careers that they pursue.

Best of luck with your exams and future careers, and – as an executive summary of Part I of this book might read – be good.

Keith Amarakone
Sukhmeet S. Panesar

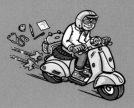

Preface

In the six years since the first editions were published, there have been many changes in medicine, and in the way it is taught. These second editions have been largely rewritten to take these changes into account, and keep *Crash Course* up to date for the twenty-first century. New material has been added to include recent research and all pharmacological and disease management information has been updated in line with current best practice. We've listened to feedback from hundreds of students who have been using *Crash Course* and have improved the structure and layout of the books accordingly: pathology material has been closely integrated with the relevant basic medical science; there are more MCQs and the clarity of text and figures is better than ever.

The principles on which we developed the series remain the same, however. Medicine is a huge subject, and the last thing a student needs when exams are looming is to waste time assembling information from different sources, and wading through pages of irrelevant detail. As before, *Crash Course* brings you all the information you need, in compact, manageable volumes that integrate basic medical science with clinical practice. We still tread the fine line between producing clear, concise text and providing enough detail for those aiming at distinction. The series is still written by medical students with recent exam experience, and checked for accuracy by senior faculty members from across the UK.

I wish you the best of luck in your future careers!

Dr Dan Horton-Szar
Series Editor (Basic Medical Sciences)

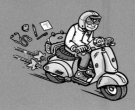

Acknowledgements

I'd like to thank all those who've helped with the writing of this book – but especially Richard, Ben, the other Ben, Sarah and Mike – whose suggestions, sensible and otherwise, have been appreciated.

KA

Firstly, my sincerest gratitude goes to my mentors, Professor Aziz Sheikh and Professor Sir Ara Darzi, individuals who have been a constant source of inspiration. I would like to thank Dr Dan Horton-Szar, Mr Mike Porter, Dr Helen Ward, Dr Gopalakrishnan Netuveli and Dr David Blane for their invaluable guidance and constructive criticism. Thanks also to Fiona Conn, Hannah Kenner and Barbara McAviney for all their assistance in overseeing the successful completion of the project. And last but not least, all my friends for their support.

SSP

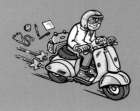

Dedications

To Ink and everyone else whose ear I bent whilst writing this, for your interest (genuine and feigned) and support, I salute you.

KA

All that I am or ever aspire to be, I owe to my mother.

SSP

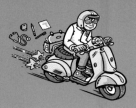

Contents

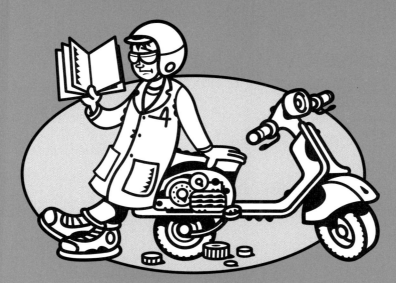

MEDICAL ETHICS AND THE LAW

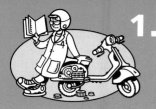

1. Principles of Ethics

Introduction to medical ethics

'Ethics' or 'moral philosophy' is the study of morals in human conduct. Like all branches of philosophy, it deals with the 'critical evaluation of assumptions and arguments' (Raphael 1981). 'Medical ethics' is the study of morals in the medical arena. In practice this means that medical ethics plays a role wherever the question 'What ought to be done?' is raised in the medical context.

Ethics deals with:
- What is right and wrong.
- What is good and bad.
- What ought and ought not to be done.

Medical ethics, therefore, critically examines the reasons that underlie any medical decision that involves these concepts.

The purpose of medical ethics is:
- To produce a rational, coherent and consistent approach to making moral decisions in medicine.
- To emphasize a reasoned approach to making moral decisions (rather than a religious, psychological or social approach).
- To ultimately produce a complete framework based on first principles that aids universal moral decision-making and is appropriate to individual situations.

The purpose of medical ethics is NOT:
- To describe the legal constraints on doctors.
- To formalize religious teaching or sentiments.
- To provide a sociological or psychological explanation for why we behave in certain ways.
- To place moral decision-making within medicine in a historical or anthropological light (Fig. 1.1).

Why is medical ethics important?

Less than a decade ago, many medical schools did not formally teach ethics. It was thought that ethical conduct would be learnt via 'osmosis' on the wards, that the student would be able to learn what was considered right and wrong by observation of senior doctors. In contrast, the explicit teaching of ethics aims to help to foster *an ability to make rational, moral decisions* – rather than to simply do things as they have been done before.

The importance of this for the medical student, in real life, and in ethics exams, is that it is not simply the conclusion you reach that is important. Rather, it is also the rigour and coherence of the arguments that lead you to your conclusion which are important.

One of the problems that dishearten medical students is that there often don't seem to be any correct answers in medical ethics. You *could* argue that abortion (or euthanasia, cloning, in vitro fertilization, dating patients and so on) is right or wrong – there seem to be arguments for both sides of the debate. However, it is important to use only those arguments that are valid or justifiable (Fig. 1.2).

Theoretical ethics

A very brief history of (Western) ethical philosophy

The tradition of ethical philosophy started with the ancient Greeks. The first important names are those of Socrates and his immediate successors – Plato and Aristotle. From there, there is a continuity in ethical discussion that can be seen through Hellenistic, Roman and medieval thought to present-day ethics.

Socrates (469–399 BC) asked 'How should a man live, in order to achieve *eudaimonia* (happiness or flourishing)?' His answer was that the good life was the one lived in accordance with *arête* (virtue).

Plato (427–347 BC) believed in the existence of a world of 'forms' beyond the material world, which is accessible only by reason. Within this world of forms exists 'perfect goodness'. Thus, Plato thought moral knowledge was coded for in the structure of the universe, in a similar way to how some

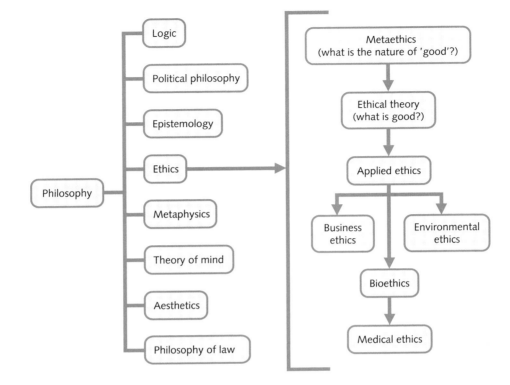

Fig. 1.1 Branches of philosophy and the position of medical ethics.

Fig. 1.2 How to write an ethics essay.

How to write an ethics essay
Make an outline/plan of the essay before writing a first draft
Answer the question: make sure that everything you say is relevant to the essay title. Ways to help you to do this include: Define how you interpret any unclear terms at the beginning of your essay State in your own words what the problem is and the issues you plan to address in your essay Briefly state the scope of the question
When making your arguments in the body of the essay, try and develop points in a logical way by: Stating your perspective and reasons for holding it Looking at opposing arguments: you must use other people's ideas as well as your own to show that you are aware of the major arguments in a certain area. Don't forget to reference other people's ideas Saying why your arguments are better/more convincing
When you re-read your first draft, decide what the 'purpose' of each paragraph is, and whether what you have written is achieving that purpose
When concluding, sum up the reasons for your argument that you have already outlined: don't include new arguments in the conclusion
No-one expects a firm conclusion: ethical debates have raged for millennia without resolution; however, you should say why you believe one argument is better than another whilst still acknowledging that both have their merits

mathematicians believe numbers are coded. So, people can 'discover' moral facts in the same way that we 'discovered' facts about geometry.

Aristotle (384–322 BC) was more practical than Plato. He believed that people were pre-programmed with the virtues, but were responsible for the degree to which they implemented them. 'Good' people choose a 'mean' between extremes and so do everything in moderation. So the virtuous man would be neither reckless (too courageous) nor timid (not courageous enough).

Epicurus (341–270 BC) considered *eudaimonia* to be equivalent to pleasure; however, even he advocated Aristotelian moderation.

The advent of Christianity saw a harmonization between Greek philosophy and Gospel teachings. St Augustine (354–430) used Plato's ideas about the nature of the 'state'. He claimed true happiness could only be achieved via the 'society' of the church, and that the state was a necessary evil; subject to corrupting influences, but useful nevertheless.

St Thomas Aquinas (1224–74) incorporated Aristotle's views into Christian theology. He thought that people should try to achieve happiness by exercising their virtues in moderation.

Machiavelli (1469–1527) is famed for writing *The Prince*, one of the first books to be banned by the Catholic Church. The importance of this work lay in its suggestion that in order to rule effectively a degree of immorality was required. Many people still believe that to be successful at politics or business you have to be unethical. It wasn't until the Utilitarians (see below) that a comprehensive format for realigning law, morality and government was suggested.

During the 17th and 18th century a debate raged about whether human nature was intrinsically good or bad. Thomas Hobbes (1588–1679) claimed that human nature leads men to lead 'solitary, poor, nasty, brutish and short' lives. In order to prevent this, people form societies, which establish laws to promote everyone's interests; this is his Social Contract Theory. Contrastingly, Jean-Jacques Rousseau (1712–78) believed that we are all born as moral beings and are corrupted by civilization.

This debate is still not settled and is now framed as the nature–nurture debate. To what degree are we able to act freely? Do our genes determine our behaviour or our sense of morality?

The ancient virtues
These included:
- Wisdom.
- Justice.
- Courage.
- Moderation.
- Piety.

Ethical theories

There are three main theories that provide frameworks around which a moral response can be structured. These are:
- Utilitarianism: a form of Consequentialism.
- Kantianism: a form of Deontology.
- Virtue theory: a form of Narrative Ethics.

Why should we bother with these theories? Can we not rely on some 'Golden principle' such as 'Do onto others as you would have them do unto you?' Perhaps such a principle is sufficient to help to guide our moral decisions on a day-to-day basis, but often it falters on *hard cases*. These are the ethical dilemmas where there is no obvious path to take. In addition, we need to provide reasons why any such golden principle is right and why others might be wrong.

However, no single theory can solve all ethical problems; in fact, we should not expect them to. The purpose of ethical theory is to help us to think more clearly about ethical problems. Part of the reason ethical dilemmas still exist is that no theory is perfect, they all have some weaknesses.

Utilitarianism (consequentialism)

Utilitarianism is often summed up as doing '*the greatest good for the greatest number*'. It is a *consequentialist* theory as it holds that the outcomes (that is, the consequences) of an action are the most morally important component of that action.

Utilitarianism was founded by Jeremy Bentham (1748–1832) and John Stuart Mill (1806–73). It is based on a single principle: the principle of utility. This holds that we ought to produce the maximum amount of utility. What then is 'utility'? There are many definitions, but most are concerned with some aspect of well-being. Bentham and Mill thought that utility was pleasure or happiness. Other utilitarians include values such as friendship, knowledge, health and beauty. Still others believe that the concept of utility is best applied to the satisfaction of preferences rather than any intrinsic values.

Bentham was a lawyer who believed that law and morality could be made rational by a scientific study of human nature. He thought that humans were governed by two factors – 'pleasure and pain' – and that it was in their nature to seek pleasure and avoid pain. For Bentham, laws were only 'good' if they maximized pleasure and minimized pain for the majority of people. The 'scientific' foundation of utilitarianism comes from the requirement to do 'happiness sums'. Bentham thought it was possible to classify how good an action is by measuring how much pleasure or pain was brought about by that action. He called this process 'felicific calculus'.

Mill differed from Bentham in two important ways:
1. He thought that cultural and spiritual pleasures should be sought in preference to physical pleasures.
2. He thought that people should ordinarily stick to moral rules rather than calculate the balance of utility for each ethical problem.

Even though Mill advocated moral rules, he is still a utilitarian, because he held that these moral rules should be calculated using the principle of utility. This is what is know as *rule utilitarianism*. For example, lying in general might produce less utility than telling the truth. Therefore, there is a rule that says 'Do not lie!' However, we could imagine a scenario where telling a particular lie might produce more utility than telling the truth would. The rule utilitarian would still tell the truth. Other utilitarians, known as *act utilitarians*, would appeal directly to the principle of utility and lie (Fig. 1.3).

The advantages of utilitarianism are that:
- It fits with two strong intuitions that:
  – morality is about promotion of well-being and
  – we should maximize well-being.
- It is a single principle that tries to deal with appropriateness of other principles, such as *always* telling the truth.
- It incorporates a principle of equality: each person's happiness is equal.
- It can be extended to the animal kingdom: some utilitarians have argued that the capacity to suffer (and feel pain) means our treatment of animals ought to be subject to moral scrutiny.

The disadvantages of utilitarianism are that:
- There are problems dealing with intuitively immoral actions: is it right to let one patient die in

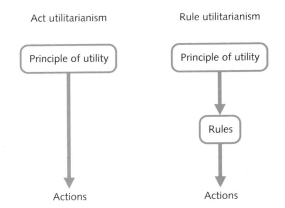

Fig. 1.3 Act v. rule utilitarianism. In act utilitarianism the principle of utility is directly used to guide actions. In rule utilitarianism the principle of utility is used to formulate general rules which in turn are used to guide actions.

order to harvest their organs and perhaps save five lives?
- Utilitarianism demands too much: in always asking us to do the *best* action, everyone is expected to be both heroic and saintly. For example, the maximizing principle demands that not only should we donate blood and bone marrow as often as we can, but also that we may well be morally obliged to donate one of our kidneys as well.
- The equality principle is overly impersonal in demanding that we treat the well-being of our friends and family as equivalent to that of strangers.
- In principle, a small increase in pleasure for the majority will override a vast degree of pain for a minority.

Utilitarianism
- Outcomes are the most important component of doing 'good'.
- 'Good' is defined in terms of 'utility'.
- Single principle = maximize utility.
- Act utilitarians act to maximize consequences all the time.
- Rule utilitarians use the principle to produce general rules that they then follow.

Kantianism (deontology)

Deontology covers those theories that emphasize moral *duties* and *rules* rather than consequences (from the Greek *deon*, meaning 'duty'). Kantianism is broadly synonymous with deontology as it is the most comprehensive example of a moral theory of this kind. However, perhaps the best *known* deontological principles are those set down in the Ten Commandments.

Kantianism takes its name from Immanuel Kant (1724–1804), a Prussian philosopher who disagreed with the utilitarians. He believed that morality was not dependent on how much happiness resulted from particular actions. Rather, he thought morality was something humans imposed upon themselves because they are rational beings. Although Christian, Kant did not believe that God was necessary for moral law.

Kant argued that we can find out which moral rules to obey by using our powers of reason. He said that by seeing whether our desires can be applied universally, we can tell whether or not they follow rational moral principles. This 'universalizability' test is called the 'categorical imperative'. It states:

> Act only on that maxim through which you can at the same time will that it should become a universal law.

This means that we should behave in such a way that we can imagine everyone can behave. For example, if our 'maxim' or 'desire' is to 'steal other people's things when we want them', we need to consider whether or not this maxim could be held for everyone. Kant said that if everyone stole things whenever they wanted, the whole notion of theft and personal property would collapse; if this happens, the concept of 'stealing' becomes illogical. The same holds for the idea of lying. Telling a lie only 'works' if there is a general belief that people tell the truth. If everyone lied whenever it might benefit them, then this general belief in truth-telling would collapse and lying would itself become pointless. Therefore, Kant said that the moral law obliges us not to steal and not to lie.

Kant also said that because humans are rational beings, we should never treat people *'simply as a means but always at the same time as an end'*. The emphasis here is on the fact that all people are equal (because they are rational) and deserve equal respect.

The advantages of Kantianism are that:

- It has a simplicity of structure: moral rules must pass the 'categorical imperative'.
- It places a special responsibility upon individuals for their actions.
- It addresses factors other than consequences, such as motives, which intuitively seem important in moral decision-making.
- It allows a certain degree of choice; if more than one option is morally acceptable, then the individual can choose which to carry out (unlike utilitarianism where the *best* option *must* be selected).

The disadvantages of Kantianism are that:

- It depends on freedom of will and rationality: are we perfectly free and rational?
- It seems to be absolutist in nature: the imperative 'do not lie' is intractable – it means 'do not lie . . . EVER', even if it prevents great harm from occurring.
- The moral rules can seem quite abstract and unable to deal with the complexities of real-life ethical dilemmas.
- Two duties (imperatives) may conflict, so what happens then?

Kantianism
- A rule-based ethical theory.
- The 'categorical imperative' is a 'universalizability' test.
- Emphasis on treating individuals as an 'end' not just a 'means'.
- Moral rules are absolute – that is they can't be broken.

Virtue theory (narrative ethics)

Virtue theory operates within a slightly different arena from both utilitarianism and Kantianism. It does not focus on either moral rules or consequences, rather it concentrates on character and motivation.

Virtue ethics is rooted in the classical Greek approach to ethics as typified by Aristotle (indeed, many virtue theorists classify themselves as neo-Aristotelians). It is the cultivation of virtue within one's character that is the function of morality. Philosophers such as Alisdair MacIntyre (b.1929) have advocated that the study of ethics should be directed towards how we ought to live our lives, and advised which ethical characteristics we should try and develop. In a sense, virtue theory tries to concentrate on what it is that makes some people 'good' or 'virtuous' and how they are different from those who are not. The right thing to do in a given dilemma is that which a 'virtuous' person would do. Virtue theory emphasizes:

- The *interpretation* of certain facts of a dilemma, within a specific *context*. That is by looking at the values pertinent to those involved in a dilemma rather than abstract hypothesizing.
- *Reasoning by analogy* rather than reasoning by deduction or from principles.

The advantages of the virtue theory are that:

- It is more personal than either utilitarianism or Kantianism: it supports those actions done out of benevolence, friendship, honesty and love in and of themselves, rather than because they are 'maximizing positive value' or are carried out in accordance with 'moral duty'.
- It is more adaptive to the particular context of a dilemma, rather than being bound by rules or applying a 'calculation' to a dilemma.

The disadvantages of the virtue theory are that:

- A list of virtues is insufficient to justify why we should promote them.
- It is unhelpful in resolving moral conflicts.
- There is no universally agreed-upon list of virtues to promote.

Virtue theory
- Concentrates on character and motivation.
- Concerned with what it is to be a good person rather than specific problems.

The four principles

In the late 1970s, two Americans, Tom Beauchamp and James Childress, introduced the idea of the 'four principles'. They are:

- Autonomy: the principle of respecting the decisions made by those capable of making decisions.
- Beneficence: the principle of providing benefits.
- Non-maleficence: the principle of avoiding doing harm.
- Justice: the principle of ensuring fairness and equity in the distribution of risks and benefits.

The four principles do not constitute an 'ethical theory' as such, rather they are guidelines: a framework around which an ethical discussion can be based (Fig. 1.4).

Autonomy

Autonomy literally means 'self-rule'. In essence it refers to an ability 1) to reason and think about one's own choices, 2) to decide how to act and 3) to act on that decision, all without hindrance from other people.

Autonomy is more than simply being free to do what one wants to do. It implies that rational thought is involved in a decision. Whilst many animals are free to do what they want, they are not autonomous because they do not critically evaluate the benefits and risks to themselves, or others, involved in their decisions.

In respecting a person's autonomy we recognize that they are entitled to make decisions that affect their own lives. Justification for this principle is most obviously found in Kantian theory: the idea that people should be treated not simply as means, but as ends in themselves. However, support for autonomy can also be found in those versions of *rule-utilitarianism* which hold that the best outcomes arise when autonomy is respected.

Beneficence and non-maleficence

Beneficence is the principle of doing 'good'. In the medical context, this generally means improving the welfare of patients. Non-maleficence involves 'not

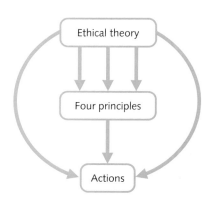

Fig. 1.4 The position of the four principles. The four principles can be thought of as a midway point between theories and actions.

harming patients'. It is associated with the Latin phrase '*primum non nocere*' or 'above all, do no harm'. As 'doing good' and 'not doing harm' seem to fall on a continuum, there is often confusion about where non-maleficence ends and beneficence begins. One way of looking at the two is to think of non-maleficence as a duty towards all people, whereas beneficence, as we can't help everyone, is a duty we choose to discharge on specific people. Medical staff, by accepting a patient, have chosen to act beneficently towards that person. The principles of beneficence and non-maleficence are broadly similar to the principle of utility. Kant also talks about the duty of beneficence: he sees this as a type of 'imperfect' duty, that is one that is subordinate to the 'perfect' duties necessitated by the categorical imperative.

Justice

The principle of justice within the medical context refers to the allocation or distribution of resources amongst the population. Basically, this principle demands the fair treatment of 'equals' within the health-care system. There is, however, no single answer as to what constitutes fair and equal distribution. The following are possible answers:

1. *Equality* – Each person receives an equal share of the resources available.
2. *Need* – Each person receives resources appropriate to how much that person needs.
3. *Desert* – Each person receives resources according to how much they deserve them (in terms of contribution, effort or merit).
4. *Desire* – Each person gets what they want. Desire forms the basis of a utilitarian outlook: it is important as it forms the basis for cost-effective analysis and quality-adjusted life years (see p. 32) (Fig. 1.5).

Oaths, declarations and rights

The Hippocratic Oath (~425 BC) was probably the first medical oath. It encourages a number of concepts that are still relevant today: the teaching of medicine, the consideration of the patient's best interests, confidentiality and the abstinence from 'whatever is deleterious and mischievous'. However, it doesn't mention concepts such as autonomy or justice, and forbids procuring abortions. The original Hippocratic oath is now rarely taken in UK medical schools.

The Declaration of Geneva (1948, revised 1968 and 1983) is a modern-day Hippocratic Oath,

Fig. 1.5 A comparison of the four principles and ethical theories.

A comparison of the four principles and ethical theories

Principle	Utilitarianism	Kantianism	Virtue theory
Respect for autonomy	This generally brings about best consequences but can be overridden	An essential component of why we should be moral – a respect for all rational (autonomous) beings	Respectfulness is consistent with virtuous behaviour
Beneficence	Maximizing good (beneficence) is the central concept	Not central – the 'right' action is the one that is one's moral duty – benevolence is not important	The principle of beneficence is equivalent to the virtue of benevolence
Non-maleficence	Can also be seen as a very utilitarian goal – minimizing harm	As above	The principle of non-maleficence is equivalent to the virtue of non-malevolence
Justice	Not necessarily concerned with the distribution of utility – simply the maximization of it	The universalizability criterion ensures a type of justice where all people are equal by virtue of their rationality	Corresponds to virtues of justice or fairness

requiring doctors to make the health of their patients their 'first consideration'.

The Declaration of Helsinki (1964, revised 1975 and 1983) deals with biomedical research. It states that 'the interests of the subject must always prevail over the interests of science and society'.

In addition, the General Medical Council (GMC) issues guidance on what it considers to be the ethical duties of British doctors. It publishes this in *Duties of a Doctor*, which covers truth-telling, confidentiality, and good medical practice in general.

Legal and moral rights

When talking about rights, it is necessary to distinguish *legal rights* from *moral rights*. Legal rights are enshrined in legislation. In the UK (where we don't have a written Constitution or Bill of Rights), legal rights are created either by Acts of Parliament or by judges in case-law. Moral rights may not have an equivalent legal right and some legal rights may not be moral rights.

Legal rights

The most important piece of legislation that deals with rights is the Human Rights Act 1998. This makes rights from the 1950 European Convention on Human Rights (ECHR) enforceable against public authorities, which includes hospitals, in England and Wales. The full extent of the power of this Act is still unknown as much of the legislation is untested in the Courts.

Some of the Articles that are important in medicine are:

Article 2: Right to Life

Everyone's right to life shall be protected by law

- Does this mean everyone is entitled to any possible treatment? Even if it is unlikely to succeed?
- Does it mean that the withholding/withdrawal of care might be unlawful? How will this affect the *Bland* case, which allowed the withdrawal of nutrition/hydration from patients in permanent vegetative states?

Article 3: Prohibition of Torture (Degrading Treatment)

No-one shall be subjected to torture or inhuman or degrading treatment or punishment

- Could this be used to challenge poor-quality treatment or failure to provide treatment within a

certain time? Does waiting 18 months for a hip replacement constitute degrading treatment? Does waiting for 24 hours on a trolley in A&E constitute degrading treatment?
- Do laws prohibiting the assisted suicide/euthanasia of terminally ill patients constitute inhuman or degrading treatment?

Article 8: Right to Respect for Private and Family Life

Everyone has the right to respect for his private and family life, his home and his correspondence

- How might this affect issues of confidentiality? For example, in genetic testing where a positive result may have implications not only for a patient, but also for their siblings and children.

Article 12: Right to Marry and Found a Family

Men and women of marriageable age have the right to marry and found a family according to the national laws governing the exercise of that right

- Could this article be used to challenge limitations on access to fertility treatment?

Moral rights
What is a moral right?

Moral rights are less easy to understand than legal rights. Part of the problem is that there still doesn't seem to be a general consensus, beyond the point that they constitute a form of deontology, as to what moral rights are. Some claim that moral rights are factual, and so can be said to be true or false. Others claim that using rights just asserts a position or feeling rather than a fact. Ronald Dworkin suggests that rights are special kinds of fact – moral facts – which act as 'trumps' in moral disputes. This way of thinking sees moral rights as 'insistent normative demands' that take precedence over other types of moral argument.

However, rights are not all of the same kind; they can be positive or negative:
- A negative right: generally confers a freedom from interference, for example the 'right to life' involves a freedom from being killed.
- A positive right: confers a duty on someone else to provide for the right holder, for example the 'right to health care' means that the government must provide hospitals, nurses and doctors to treat citizens.

An introduction to medical law

The UK legal system has two equal *sources* of law: parliament and the courts:

- Parliament-made law consists of Acts and Statutes.
- Court-made law is described as Common Law.

The courts are able to interpret statutes, but not overturn them. In contrast, parliament can over-rule judge-made decisions.

Criminal/civil law

The UK legal system also has two *types* of law: criminal and civil law. Both types of law involve one party being injured by another. However, in general, criminal law deals with cases where the injury is considered to be severe enough for the state to have an interest in preventing or protecting the public from it. In civil (Tort) law, where one person is wronged by another, the aggrieved party takes the wrongdoer to court in order to receive compensation.

In criminal law:

- Cases are described as *R v. Smith* (that is 'The Queen and Smith').
- A defendant is accused of committing a crime by the prosecution.
- Proof must be 'beyond reasonable doubt'.

In civil law:

- Cases are described as *Smith v. Jones* (that is 'Smith and Jones').
- The defendant is being sued by the plaintiff (the injured party).
- Proof must be 'on the balance of probabilities'.

Most medical law cases are brought within the civil-justice system (rather than the criminal). Most of these cases are brought under the tort (or wrong) of negligence. However, in extreme cases health-care professionals can be charged with criminal offences including battery and assault.

Medical negligence

There are five basic components of a medical negligence action:

1. A duty of care: it must be shown that the defendant (that is the person or authority accused of negligence) owed the plaintiff (that is the injured party or the person accusing the defendant of negligence) a duty of care:
   A. English law does not impose upon doctors a duty to provide treatment to whoever requires it (in contrast to the situation in France where Good Samaritan Laws exist) except when:
      i. A patient presents to an A&E department.
      ii. When a GP is requested to provide emergency treatment to a person in his practice area.
   B. The duty of care of a GP crystallizes when the patient:
      i. Registers with that GP and then,
      ii. Consults with the GP on the occasion in question.
   C. The duty of care of a hospital doctor crystallizes when the patient is formally accepted into hospital.
2. A standard of care: there must be a standard of care that could be expected from the defendant – this is normally the standard of reasonable care – that is the level of care that could be expected from an ordinary member of that branch of medicine:
   A. The standard of care doctors are expected to reach was asserted by the case *Bolam v. Friern Hospital Management Committee* [1957] 1 WLR 582. The standard of care was set as that of 'the ordinary skilled man exercising and professing to have that special skill'.
   B. This standard has become known as the Bolam Test – it is applicable to all aspects of treatment, diagnosis, the disclosure of information or risks to patients.
3. A breach: the plaintiff must show that the defendant did not reach a reasonable standard of care.
4. Causation: the plaintiff must then show that that breach caused the damage they claim to have suffered: the test used to prove causation is often referred to as the '*but for*' test. It says the plaintiff must demonstrate that *but for* the defendant's negligence, he would not have suffered the harm in respect of which he seeks damages.
5. Damages: some level of damage must have occurred to the plaintiff. The purpose of bringing an action is to gain compensation for damages; if no damages have occurred, there is little point in bringing an action.

- What is the purpose of medical ethics?
- What is normative ethics?
- Who was Bentham?
- 'The greatest good for the greatest number' summarizes which theory?
- What are the differences between utilitarianism and Kantianism?
- What is the categorical imperative?
- Reasoning by analogy is a characteristic of which theory?
- What are the four principles?
- What does the Declaration of Helsinki cover?
- How might Article 2: The Right to Life, of the Human Rights Act 1998 affect the provision of medical treatment in England and Wales?
- Name a positive right.
- Name a negative right.

References

Raphael DD 1981 Moral Philosophy. Oxford: Oxford
  University Press

Further reading

Gillon R 1986 Philosophical Medical Ethics. Chichester: John
  Wiley & Sons
Harris J 1985 The Value of Life. London: Routledge & Kegan
  Paul
Kagan S 1998 Normative Ethics. Oxford: Westview Press

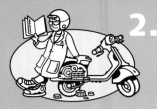

2. Professional Ethics

❝ When God said that lying was a sin, he made an exception for doctors, and he gave them permission to lie as many times a day as they saw patients.

Dumas

When Dumas wrote the above, it was probably meant to be slightly ironic. However, it does reflect the historical notion that the extent to which patients are told the truth was a matter for the doctor to decide. The Hippocratic Oath is notably silent on the issue of telling patients the truth. In fact, Hippocrates advised the physician to 'calmly and adroitly conceal most things from their patients . . . turning his attention away from what is being done to him . . . revealing nothing of the patient's future or present condition'. So from ancient times until comparatively recently, lying to patients was not necessarily disapproved of, or even discouraged. Indeed 'to lie like a physician' used to be a compliment!

Current thought is completely different. The General Medical Council (GMC) states that doctors have a duty to be 'honest and trustworthy'. The Bristol Royal Inquiry made 37 recommendations on how a greater culture of respect and honesty could be fostered within the NHS.

Withholding the truth includes:
- Outright lies.
- Temporary deception.
- Not answering direct questions.
- Giving false hope.

Telling the truth

The concept of 'telling the truth' has two facets:
1. The 'telling' part, which deals with the *communication* of information.

   and

2. The 'truth' part, which holds that the information given has to be *true*.

From an ethical perspective, truthful information is important for a number of reasons:
- For reasons of autonomy; truthful information helps patients to decide how to proceed with treatment.
- Even if the information doesn't lead to a treatment decision, the patient may still wish to know information about their health, because their health is intricately linked with their sense of self.
- For reasons of trust, it is generally accepted that truth-telling promotes a sense of trust between both the doctor and their patient, and in general between doctors and the public at large.

So, it seems that in general, truth-telling is a necessary duty. However, is it an absolute one? Are there any circumstances in which it might be okay to lie to patients? What about not telling the *whole* truth? Is there a difference between avoiding answering a direct question, and telling a lie? The following scenarios illustrate the general principles at stake.

Scenario 1

A patient, Mrs X, is brought to A&E after being caught in a house fire. Mrs X's three children were also in the fire; two have died and it is not known whether the other will survive or not. Mrs X herself is in a critical condition. Mrs X asks you, the doctor treating her, how her children are.

You suspect that telling the truth will distress her so much that it may well lead to her death. Do you deceive her for a short period of time?

Here we have a conflict of ethical principles:
1. Respect for autonomy holds we should not lie to our patient.
2. Beneficence holds that lying may be crucial in saving the patient's life.

The conflict in principles is mirrored by a conflict in different ethical theories as well: utilitarianism would tell us to lie, Kantianism would oblige us to tell the truth. How can a compromise be reached?

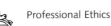

Mrs X has asked a direct question and an ill-thought-out answer could be fatal to her. Ideally, we would like to be able to reassure Mrs X without lying to her. Deflecting her questions may be difficult. The bad news needs to be communicated to her, but is perhaps best done when her own medical condition is more stable.

It has been suggested that lying to patients is justified only 'if a person, acting rationally, were presented with the alternatives, he or she would always choose being lied to' (Gert & Culver 1979). The suggestion here is that when trying to promote autonomy, what is necessary is more than a simple presentation of potential options, because the way in which the options are presented may affect the ability of Mrs X to make an autonomous choice.

Scenario 2

Mr Y has a poor (but not terminal) prognosis due to cancer. You are treating Mr Y, and are about to tell him his diagnosis and prognosis.

Before you do so, his son, a local GP, who has guessed the diagnosis, urges you not to tell his father the truth. The son explains that his mother, Mr Y's wife, died a mere two months ago of a very aggressive cancer, and he fears that if his father knows the truth, he will 'give in' because the father thinks that any diagnosis of cancer is one without hope of recovery.

In this scenario, the deception is not a short-term one to allow recovery, but a permanent one. However, the conflict of principles is similar: autonomy vs. beneficence.

Weighing up the two sides of the equation is difficult because there are two ideas, or conceptions, about the nature of autonomy:

- One view is that autonomy is about *making decisions*: being in charge of one's own destiny.
- A different view is that autonomy is about making *certain types* of decision: specifically the types of decision that are consistent with a general life-plan or goal.

These differing conceptions of autonomy are developed further in the section on paternalism.

Telling the truth and the law

The legal implications of truth-telling mainly concern whether or not the consent given is valid. In order for consent to be valid, it must be *informed consent*. The law tends to consider whether doctors have fully disclosed risks inherent in treatment before obtaining consent.

There are different conceptions of autonomy:
- Long-term autonomy: value lies in promoting life-long goals that are consistent with deeply held and considered beliefs and values.
- Short-term autonomy: value lies in being able to make decisions about one's own health care – whether rationally based or capricious.

Your views on which conception of autonomy you consider to be more important may shape whether or not you believe that deceiving patients can ever be morally acceptable.

The important cases that dealt with disclosure of risk are:

1. *Chatterton v. Gerson* [1981] 1 All ER 257
2. *Sidaway v. Board of Governors of the Bethlem Royal Hospital and the Maudsley Hospital* [1985] 1 All ER 643

In *Chatterton v. Gerson*, the courts looked at when doctors who didn't disclose risks would be guilty of trespass to the person. They said that:

> . . . once the patient is informed in broad terms of the nature of the procedure which is intended, and gives her consent, that consent is real, and the cause of the action on which to base a claim for failure to go into risks and implications is negligence, not trespass.

The key phrase from this judgement is that patients need to be informed '*in broad terms of the nature of the procedure*'. If this is done, then the charge of trespass, or battery, cannot be brought.

The courts also looked at when a non-disclosure of risks could lead to a charge of negligence. They said that a doctor:

> . . . ought to warn what may happen by misfortune however well the operation is done, if there is a real risk of a misfortune inherent in the operation.

The key phrase here is that doctors 'ought to warn . . . if there is a *real* risk'.

Who decides what constitutes a real risk was looked at in the *Sidaway* case. The outcome of this case was an endorsement of the *Bolam Test* (as discussed in Consent section). This test holds that in questions of disclosure of risks, a doctor is only negligent if there is no reasonable body of medical practice that would have made the same choice. Effectively, this means that the medical profession itself sets the standards for disclosure of risk.

A popular rule of thumb is to disclose risks that are greater than 1%. BUT, if there is a grave risk (such as death or permanent disability), especially for minor procedure, then this 1% rule doesn't hold, and risks with a probability of less than 1% must also be disclosed. However, the doctor is duty-bound to answer any question truthfully. This is even more important if the procedure is a non-therapeutic one, or safer alternatives exist.

Other countries have developed different tests:
- Australia has a *prudent-patient* test: here a doctor must disclose those risks that a prudent patient would wish to know.
- Japan supports a *therapeutic privilege* where doctors don't need to disclose risks (or even a diagnosis) if they believe it isn't in the patient's best interests.

- To avoid a charge of trespass to the person, the doctor must inform the patient of the '*broad terms of the nature of the procedure*'.
- To avoid a charge of negligence, the doctor must inform the patient '*if there is a real risk*' of harm.
- What constitutes a '*real risk*' is set by a degree of consensus within the medical profession.

Informed consent and its elements

Treatment without consent can lead to the health-care practitioner being liable for trespass to the person, negligence or, in extreme cases, a criminal prosecution of assault or battery.

These legal provisions mean that patients can veto care. Treatment can only be forced upon patients in narrowly defined circumstances. Consent is not required when:
- The patient is unconscious and requires *emergency* treatment.

- Testing for certain infectious diseases: these include the 'notifiable' diseases of cholera, plague, relapsing fever, smallpox and typhus.
- The patient is incapable of giving consent, for example in cases of mental disability (see p. 52) or a young child (see p. 49).

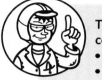

The components of a valid consent
- Being informed.
- Capacity.
- Voluntariness.
- Making a decision.

Informed consent (also see 'Telling the truth and the law')

The charge of battery can be brought against a doctor in the following situations:
1. Where no consent has been obtained.
2. When force is used.
3. When the treatment carried out is entirely different from the one specified.

Most charges are of negligence: for failure to warn the patient of risks. The courts determine which risks need to be mentioned to patients by using the *Bolam Test*. This test derives from the case of *Bolam v. Friern Hospital Management Committee* [1957] 1 WLR 582.

John Bolam was a psychiatric patient undergoing electro-convulsive therapy (ECT). He was not warned of a risk of fractures due to the convulsions, nor was he given muscle relaxants, or manually restrained. As a result of the ECT, he sustained bilateral fractures of the acetabula.

The judge defined the test of negligence to be: 'the standard of the ordinary skilled man exercising and professing to have that special skill'. Because other doctors testified that they would have treated Bolam in the same way that he was treated, that is, a '*reasonable body*' of medical practitioners would not have done anything differently, Bolam's doctor was found not guilty of negligence.

The Bolam Test originally applied to all aspects of treatment and diagnosis. It was applied to warning of risks by a subsequent case, that of *Sidaway v. Board of Governors of the Bethlem Royal Hospital and the Maudsley Hospital* [1985] 1 All ER 643.

The standard of negligence was set out by the case of *Bolam v. Friern Hospital Management Committee* [1957] 1 WLR 582. It requires the standard of care not to fall below: 'the standard of the ordinary skilled man exercising and professing to have that special skill'. Effectively, this standard is set by the medical profession.

Guidelines for obtaining informed consent

The GMC has detailed 12 key pieces of information to give to patients in order to obtain informed consent:

1. Details of the diagnosis, and prognosis, and the likely prognosis if the condition is left untreated.
2. Uncertainties about the diagnosis including options for further investigation prior to treatment.
3. Options for treatment or management of the condition, including the option not to treat.
4. The purpose of a proposed investigation or treatment; details of the procedures or therapies involved, including subsidiary treatment such as methods of pain relief; how the patient should prepare for the procedure; and details of what the patient might experience during or after the procedure including common and serious side effects.
5. For each option, explanations of the likely benefits and the probabilities of success; and discussion of any serious or frequently occurring risks, and of any lifestyle changes that may be caused by, or necessitated by, the treatment.
6. Advice about whether a proposed treatment is experimental.
7. How and when the patient's condition and any side effects will be monitored or reassessed.
8. The name of the doctor who will have overall responsibility for the treatment and, where appropriate, names of the senior members of his or her team.
9. Whether doctors in training will be involved, and the extent to which students may be involved in an investigation or treatment.

10. A reminder that patients can change their mind about a decision at any time.
11. A reminder that patients have a right to seek a second opinion.
12. Where applicable, details of costs or charges which the patient may have to meet.

Remember: when presenting information to the patient, it must be at an appropriate level. Valid consent can only be given if the patient can understand the information. The following may help when presenting information:

1. Provide information in the patient's own language: this may involve the use of a professional interpreter or a member of the patient's family. Remember, however, the patient will have to consent to the use of this person. (This applies to spoken languages and sign-language.)
2. Use leaflets: these can be given to the patient to go away and read. They should be given an opportunity to ask any questions the leaflets may have raised. Ensure the leaflets are current.
3. Use diagrams: the patient may not know where her pancreas is; drawing even a simple diagram of where it is in relation to the rest of her organs, and of the position of a surgical scar, can be helpful.
4. Ask the patient if they would like a family member or friend to be present.
5. Ask if the patient would like to tape-record the consultation.
6. If the consultation involves breaking bad news, do it in a sensitive way. It may also be helpful to inform the patient of counselling services and/or patient support groups if appropriate.
7. Encourage input from other members of the health-care team. Patients may more readily understand information from nurses, simply because they may feel less nervous or less embarrassed around them.
8. Answer patients' questions directly, don't be evasive.
9. Allow plenty of time to understand the information given.

Capacity to consent (competence)

Capacity refers to the ability of an individual to make decisions with respect to their medical treatment. It is presumed, in the absence of evidence to the contrary, that adult patients are capable of giving consent.

The definition of capacity has been given by the High Court in the case *Re C (Adult: Refusal of Treatment)* [1994] 1 All ER 819.

C was an inpatient at Broadmoor Prison Hospital, diagnosed with paranoid schizophrenia. C believed he was an internationally renowned doctor. C developed gangrene on the toes of one foot. C's surgeon believed C should have a below-knee amputation, but C refused, believing it better to die with both feet than live with one. C's solicitor applied for an injunction to prevent amputation, which was granted, as the courts found that, not withstanding his schizophrenia, C was capable.

The test used in this case to determine the capacity of C has become known as the *Re C Test*.

The *Re C Test* has three stages:

1. Can the patient take in and retain information?
2. Does the patient believe this information?
3. Can the patient weigh that information balancing risks and needs?

Remember: in adults, competence is a test for a minimal level of ability to use information given to weigh risks and benefits; it is *not* specific to the decision being made. In children, however, a patient's capacity may vary with the gravity of the decision involved. Different levels of competence are required for different procedures. A child may have the requisite capacity to agree to a broken wrist being plastered, but not to consent to treatment for leukaemia.

Where there is *fluctuating capacity* in an adult, capacity when the patient is at their most lucid should be determined. (This is different in children – see Chapter 3.)

Voluntary consent

For consent to be valid, it ought to be free from coercion. Whilst patients may take into account the advice of others – including medical staff, friends, family, police, prison authorities, employers and insurance companies – they must still feel that they are able to make an autonomous decision. Consent given under duress is invalid.

The courts have broadly backed this approach. They have found that consent may be invalidated if obtained fraudulently, by force or by undue influence (see *Re T* [1992] 3 WLR 782 below). Furthermore, if an adult patient refuses to give consent, the courts have held that no-one else is in a position to give proxy consent (see *F v. West Berkshire Health Authority* [1989] 2 All ER 545 below).

T [1992] 3 WLR 782, 4 All ER 649

T was pregnant and involved in a car accident. She went into premature labour and needed a caesarean section. Prior to the operation, T had a conversation with her mother. T's mother was a Jehovah's Witness, although T was not.

Subsequent to her conversation with her mother, T told hospital staff she did not want a blood transfusion. She had not indicated any concern about a transfusion earlier on.

The caesarean section was carried out without the need for a blood transfusion, although the baby was stillborn.

After the operation, T's condition deteriorated and she was admitted to ICU. It was decided that without a blood transfusion she would die.

The court of appeal decided:

- The refusal for a blood transfusion during a caesarean section might not apply to the new situation – by which point T was incapable of giving consent.
- That T had been unduly influenced by her mother's religious views, and this prevented her refusal being valid.

In this case, Lord Justice Staughton expressed a test for undue influence, saying:

> In order for an apparent consent or refusal of consent to be less than a true consent or refusal, there must be such a degree of external influence as to persuade the patient to depart from her own wishes, to an extent that the law regards it as undue.

F v. West Berkshire Health Authority [1989] 2 All ER 545

F was a 36-year-old woman, with a mental age of 5. F was a long-term resident of a mental hospital, and had formed a sexual relationship with a male resident.

F's mother and doctors thought that F ought to be sterilized.

The courts stated that:

- For a patient of adult age, no-one could give proxy consent.
- In the case of an incompetent patient, doctors could only act *in the best interests* of their patient.
- The 'best interests' would be decided on whether the doctor acted *in accordance with a responsible and competent body of relevant professionals* – that is, in accordance with the *Bolam Test* (see section on informed consent).

What are a patient's 'best interests'? (see also 'Mental disorders and competence to consent')

How do doctors, or the courts, decide what an incompetent patient's best interests are? The courts themselves have not given a clear definition of 'best interests' (Fig. 2.1). However, the Draft Mental Incapacity Bill (2003) included the following points that should be considered:

- Whether the person is likely to have capacity in relation to the matter in question in the future.
- The need to permit and encourage the person to participate, or improve their ability to participate, as fully as possible in any act done for and any decision affecting that person.
- That person's past and present wishes, feelings and those factors that the person would consider if they were able to do so.
- The views of those caring for the person or interested in their welfare.
- The views of any person granted lasting power of attorney by the now incapacitated person.
- The views of any court appointed deputy for the incapacitated person.

Clinical dilemma

You are a clinical medical student. Your consultant asks you to do a per rectum examination on an anaesthetized patient in theatre. You don't know whether the patient has consented to a student doing this. What do you do? The key points to this dilemma are:

- Consent.
- Intimate examinations.

All examinations are in a sense 'intimate' because they involve a touching of the patient. Consent should be obtained for *all* examinations. However, some examinations involve a greater invasion of personal space and, therefore, can be seen to require a greater degree of rigour in obtaining consent. The fact that anaesthetized patients are temporarily unable to give consent does not mean that students can proceed with an intimate examination.

The only time that doctors (or medical students) can perform an examination on an anaesthetized patient that has not been consented to is when such an examination would be in the best interests of the

Fig. 2.1 A summary of consent (see p. 49 for consent in children).

A summary of consent

Age Group	Who can consent to treatment		Who can refuse treatment	
>18 years	*Patients*	Yes	*Patients*	Yes
	Parents	No	*Parents*	No
	Courts	No – unless patient is incompetent, then courts can decide what is in the patient's *best interests*	*Courts*	Yes
	Doctors	No – unless patient is incompetent, then doctors can treat in the patient's *best interests*. If the doctors are unclear as to what a patient's best interests are, they can refer the decision to the courts	*Doctors*	Yes – doctors retain the right not to treat patients if they believe this is in the best interests of the patient or they have a conscientious objection (in which case they should refer to another doctor). Doctors must treat in emergencies (if in the patient's best interests)

patient. Examination by a student is most often simply for the educational benefit to that student. The doctor will perform the same examination in order to make a diagnosis. Therefore, the examination by the student will rarely be in the best interests of the patient.

If a student examines an anaesthetized patient without having first got consent, then they are liable to a charge of assault. The doctor supervising the student will also be liable to a charge of assault. Best practice in this kind of scenario would involve:

- Seeing the patient prior to surgery and obtaining consent to perform any examination.
- Informing the patient that the examination is for your education.
- Informing the patient that the examination will be repeated by the doctor.
- Informing the patient that you will be supervised by the doctor whilst performing the examination.
- Informing the patient that they can refuse to be examined by students and that this refusal will not affect their medical care.

Intimate examinations
These include examinations of the:
- Breasts.
- Groin.
- Rectum.
- Vagina.
- Male genitalia.

Paternalism in medicine

Paternalism refers to those practices and actions when 'those in positions of authority refuse to act according to people's wishes, or they restrict people's freedom, or in other ways attempt to influence their behaviour, allegedly in the recipients' own best interest' (Häyry 1998).

Medical paternalism occurs when a doctor makes a decision that he/she believes is in his/her patient's best interest but that is contrary to the wishes of a competent patient.

Remember: the notion of beneficence (doing good) involves acting so as to serve the patient's best interests. Beneficence may slide into paternalism where a doctor believes he/she is 'doing good' and

acts against the immediate wishes of the patient, or indeed without even consulting the patient.

The notion of autonomy began to gain prevalence only in the 1950s and 1960s. The traditional doctor–patient relationship was one based on the idea of the doctor furthering patient interests. It was assumed that it was in the patient's interest – indeed it was the patient's role – to be cured by the doctor. Furthermore, it was assumed that this required the patient to entrust their care to the doctor entirely.

Over the last few decades there has been a shift in attitudes where doctors are seen as being in a partnership with their patients and other health-care professionals – all working together.

The arguments *for* paternalism:
1. Doctors have a duty to act in the patient's best interests, even if the patient doesn't know what her best interests are.
2. Patients are incapable of making medical decisions because they are too technical.
3. By 'shouldering the burden' of difficult decisions, doctors are able to maximize utility.

The arguments *against* paternalism:
1. Patients are better placed than their doctors in deciding what is in their own interests. Whilst doctors may be able to make better 'medical' decisions, they are not necessarily able to make better 'moral' decisions.
2. Technical explanations can be explained to patients – given time and appropriate communication skills.
3. From a practical point of view it is difficult to show that this is true. It is plausible that total welfare may be increased by certain paternalistic actions but it is hard to prove. Once again the patient is better placed to decide what level of information they wish to be provided with.

Clinical dilemma
Paternalism: what happens when the patient doesn't want to know the diagnosis? Key points would include:
- Autonomy.
- The right not to know.
- Withholding of information.

What should happen if a patient expresses a desire not to know their diagnosis, or details of treatment? This sort of scenario may occur in a number of different settings: patients may not wish to confront a diagnosis of cancer, HIV, or genetic disease.

Scenario

Jane is 63 years of age, and is found to have an abnormality on a mammogram. Both Jane's mother and sister died of breast cancer. Jane says to her doctor: 'Please don't tell me if it's cancer, I don't want to know. Just do what you have to do.'

What to do when a patient doesn't want to know their diagnosis is a genuine moral dilemma, because it complicates our idea of autonomy. How can a patient make an autonomous decision not to know information about their health status, when that knowledge is necessary to make autonomous decisions? Can a patient give informed consent to surgery if they don't know that the proposed operation is to remove a tumour? How can an oncologist discuss options such as radiotherapy, as opposed to chemotherapy, if the patient doesn't want to know they have cancer? How in fact can the patient remain in ignorance at all if to be treated they need to go to the oncology department for that treatment?

The ethical issues in this scenario revolve around whether autonomy and a right to self-determination confer a right not to know, or a right to remain in ignorance.

Remember: if the patient asks not to be informed about their own health status, and for the doctor to go ahead and 'do what they think is best', then strictly speaking, the doctor is *not* acting paternalistically. Paternalism involves acting contrary to the patient's wishes.

The alleged 'right not to know' is somewhat problematic. It can be argued that to be meaningful a 'right to know' implies that right can be waived, so there is a complementary 'right not to know'. Others have argued that 'a *right* not to know' is too strong a term to use (remember in Chapter 1, rights were described as 'insistent normative demands', which can 'trump' other forms of moral argument) and the debate ought to be framed in terms of freedoms. So, patients may be 'free not to know', but this freedom should be weighed against the interests and concerns of others, such as the doctor's right not to make those decisions that properly belong to the patient. Of course, this does not mean that unwanted information *must* be forced upon the patient, merely that the doctor is under no obligation not to withhold the diagnosis. So:

- It remains controversial as to whether autonomy confers a right not to know.
- It is not paternalistic to withhold information if the patient has chosen to remain in ignorance about their condition.

- If you are asked to withhold information by your patient, doing so may be morally *permissible*, but not necessarily morally *compulsory*.

Confidentiality

> Whatever, in connection with my professional practice . . . I see or hear, in the life of men, which ought not to be spoken of abroad, I will not divulge, as reckoning that all such should be kept secret.
> Hippocratic Oath ~425 BC

Confidentiality has, since the time of Hippocrates, played an important role in maintaining the doctor–patient relationship. A modern version of the Hippocratic Oath is found in the Geneva Declaration, which states: 'I will respect the secrets which are confided in me, even after the patient has died.' Both the public and members of the medical profession recognize that without confidentiality health care will inevitably suffer.

The GMC asserts that a duty of confidentiality arises from a combination of:
- Patient's rights: 'Patients have a right to expect that information about them will be held in confidence by their doctors.'
and
- Consequentialist reasoning: 'Confidentiality is central to trust between doctors and patients. Without assurances about confidentiality, patients may be reluctant to give doctors the information they need in order to provide good care.'

The right to confidentiality derives ultimately from a right to autonomy. Part of self-determination is deciding who knows what about oneself. Medical consultations consist in a disclosure of information to a health-care professional. The purpose of such information is to treat the patient – it has not been given for any other reason. That information in a sense 'belongs' to the person who disclosed it and ought not to be broadcast to third parties without specific consent. If a health-care professional does not treat patients as autonomous, she is not treating them as equals – in the sense of being rational beings in control of their own lives. The importance of privacy, and by extension confidentiality, is that it forms an intimate part of who we are. Without privacy our very identities would be radically different.

The practice of keeping medical information confidential can also be supported by, or derived from, consequentialist reasoning. Justice Clark gave the following reasons for maintaining medical confidentiality in an important American case (see discussion of *Tarasoff v. Regents of the University of California*, 17 Cal. 3d 425 in Chapter 3):

1. *Deterrence from treatment* – without the assurance of confidentiality, 'those requiring treatment will be deterred from seeking assistance'.
2. *Full disclosure* – the 'guarantee of confidentiality is essential in eliciting the full disclosure necessary for effective treatment'.
3. *Successful treatment* – confidentiality is an integral part of procuring a successful treatment – trust between patient and physician or therapist is essential.

Confidentiality
When thinking about or discussing confidentiality, it is helpful to think in terms of three categories:

1. *A theoretical basis* for confidentiality – such as the right to privacy and the consequential benefits of maintaining such a system.
2. *Professional regulation*, which can include a system of oaths (e.g. the Hippocratic Oath) or guidelines from the Royal Colleges or the 'Duties of a Doctor' as laid down by the GMC.
3. *Legal regulation*, which asserts where a common law duty to maintain confidentiality exists and when it can be broken (e.g. Prevention of Terrorism Act 1989).

When can confidential information be disclosed?

The GMC has outlined that confidential information about a patient can be disclosed:

- With the patient's consent (or the consent of a person properly authorized to act on the patient's behalf, e.g. the parent of a young child).
- Within teams:
  - in order to provide best care possible
  - patient should be informed so as to understand why and when information may be shared between team members
  - when disclosure is required for a procedure that has been agreed to, *explicit* consent would not be required, for example giving relevant clinical information to the radiologist when sending a patient for an X-ray
  - in an emergency if a patient is unable to give consent, but disclosure would be in the patient's best interests

  It must be noted, however, that:
  - if a patient does not wish you to share particular information with team members, you must respect those wishes
  - it is the responsibility of *all* members of the team to ensure that other team members understand and observe confidentiality.

- To employers and insurance companies only with the patient's *written* consent. The purpose of the consultation (if on behalf of a third party) should be made clear from the outset.
- For the purpose of education, audit or research:
  - inform patient of the purpose of disclosure and that the person given access to the records will be under a duty of confidentiality, and seek their consent
  - as far as possible anonymize the data
  - keep the disclosures to the minimum necessary
  - where research projects are using identifying information, and it is not practicable to inform patients, then this needs to be brought to the attention of a research ethics committee
  - express consent should be obtained before publishing case histories and photos (many journals now require written consent from the patient).
- In the patient's best interest:
  - if a patient is unable to give consent owing to immaturity, illness or mental incapacity; however the patient should as far as possible be informed of your intention
  - if a patient is a victim of neglect, physical or sexual abuse *and* unable to give valid consent, *and* you believe disclosure will prevent further harm, you should disclose information to the *appropriate* responsible person or statutory agency.
- In the interests of others:
  - if not doing so will lead to a risk of serious harm or death (e.g. contact tracing in HIV); however,

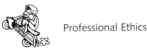
you should inform the patient of your intention to make the disclosure
- if a colleague, who is also a patient, is placing patients at risk
- if disclosure is required for the prevention or detection of a serious crime.
- When it is required by statute or the courts:
  - for example there is requirement by statute to give information under the Public Health (Infectious Diseases) Regulations SI 1988/1546 about certain 'notifiable' diseases [Remember that HIV is *not* a notifiable disease]
  - if ordered to disclose by a judge or the coroner
  - doctors are allowed to object to disclosure if an attempt is made to obtain information about those not involved in a particular proceeding or if irrelevant details are requested.
- After a patient's death:
  - the obligation of confidentiality in general persists after the patient's death
  - there are some instances when disclosure is appropriate. For example, in order to assist a coroner, as part of National Confidential enquiries or other clinical audits, on death certificates, or to obtain information relating to public health surveillance.
- To the Driver and Vehicle Licensing Agency (DVLA):
  - the DVLA is responsible for deciding if a person is medically unfit to drive
  - if a patient has a condition that impairs their ability to drive, you should explain to them that they have a legal duty to inform the DVLA
  - if the patient cannot understand this advice, for example owing to dementia, you should inform the DVLA
  - if patients refuse to accept your diagnosis, you should advise them to seek a second opinion and refrain from driving until that time
  - if a patient continues to drive when they are not fit to do so, you should make every effort to persuade them to stop; this can include telling their next of kin
  - if they cannot be persuaded, you should inform the medical advisor at the DVLA. Inform the patient that this is your intention and write to confirm that a disclosure has been made.

Legal regulation of confidentiality

This duty of confidentiality in common law arises where 'information comes to the knowledge of a

- Although the GMC Guidelines are not legally binding, they are relied upon in court so have a 'quasi-legal' status.
- There exists a key principle that confidentiality *ought* to be maintained, so if doctors make a disclosure, they must be prepared to justify why they did so.

person . . . in circumstances where he has notice, or is held to have agreed, that the information is confidential'. Such a duty is held to apply to doctors.

In addition, the Data Protection Act 1998 provides a statutory duty to maintain the confidentiality of medical records.

The Health and Social Care Act 2001 deals with the regulation of patient information. It allows the Secretary of State to make provision for the disclosure of information in the interests of improving patient care or in the public interest. In particular this allows for the disclosure of patient records to the patient or a prescribed individual on behalf of the patient.

However, there are a number of exceptions to the common law duty of confidentiality (Fig. 2.2). These include:

1. Disclosure in court, for example when a doctor is brought to give evidence on the extent or cause of an injury.
2. If the police request access to records in accordance with the Police and Criminal Evidence Act 1984.
3. 'Notifiable' disease must be reported to the authorities in accordance with the Public Health (Infectious Diseases) Regulations 1988 (SI1988, No. 1546). These include, amongst others, cholera, meningitis, anthrax, diphtheria, measles, mumps, rubella, and tuberculosis (neither HIV nor AIDS is a notifiable disease).
4. In accordance with the Prevention of Terrorism (Temporary Provisions) Act 1989.
5. The Children Act 1989 holds that information pertaining to child abuse must be given if requested by the local authority – it does not oblige doctors to report suspected abuse, although both the GMC and the BMA advise reporting.

Guidance on when doctors should or should not breach confidentiality

When doctors should not breach confidentiality:

For amusement or in conversation

To prevent a minor crime – this would probably include most instances of burglary and property-related crime

To prevent minor harm to someone else

Doctors working in a genitourinary clinic should not provide information to a third party that might identify a patient examined or treated for any sexually transmitted disease (with a few exceptions mentioned below)

To insurers, employers or any other third party without the patient's consent – preferably written

When doctors should breach confidentiality:

Notifiable diseases

Termination of pregnancy

Births

Deaths

To the police on request, e.g. name and address of driver who has committed an offence

Search warrant signed by a judge

Under court orders

When doctors have discretion:

Sharing information with the rest of the health-care team

Patients who continue to drive, but are not medically fit to do so (GMC advises disclosure)

When a third party is at significant risk

The detection or prevention of serious crime

Source: adapted from Hope T, Salvulescu J, Hendrick J 2003 Medical Ethics and Law: the core curriculum. Edinburgh: Churchill Livingstone

Patients' access to health-care records

This is governed by the Data Protection Act 1998. It applies to both computer records and paper records. It outlines eight principles of the act that ensure that:

- Information is processed fairly and lawfully.
- Information is obtained for specified and lawful purposes.
- Information is adequate, relevant and not excessive in relation to the purpose for which obtained.
- Information is accurate and, where necessary, kept up to date.
- Information is not kept for longer than necessary.
- Information is not used in ways contrary to the rights of the data subject (the patient in medical records).
- Appropriate measures are taken to prevent unauthorized disclosure of information.
- Information is not transferred to areas that cannot provide the above assurances.

The Data Protection Act 1998 gives the patient a certain number of rights with respect to their medical records. These include:

- *The right to be informed* about what information is being held, and why.
- *The right of access to personal data*. Patients have a right to a copy of their medical records. They also have the right to have this information communicated to them in a way they can understand it. However, in order to obtain this information, the patient must make a written

request, and may be required to pay a fee (not exceeding a maximum).

- *The right to correct information that is inaccurate.* If a patient feels that the information about them is misleading, they can ask for it to be changed.
- *The right to seek damages as a result of misleading information.*

Clinical dilemma

An HIV-positive patient demands you tell no-one else of his diagnosis, including others of the health-care team. Key points would include:

- Confidentiality.
- Preventing risk to third parties.

What makes HIV/AIDS different from other diseases is that there is still no cure for the disease, that patients can live apparently unaffected for a long period of time (but still be infective) and that there is a degree of stigma associated with the disease.

The ethical thinking behind maintaining confidentiality and not disclosing includes:

- The right to privacy, based on a respect for autonomy.
- The fact that the erosion of confidence in the medical consultation will lead to worse consequences (for example fewer people with HIV seeking treatment).

Factors that might persuade us in this case to break confidentiality would include:

- Not disclosing the patient's HIV status to others (including the patient's partner and potentially other health-care professionals) would mean their being unaware of an increased risk of infection.
- Not telling other members of the health-care team (e.g. the GP) may lead to the provision of inappropriate treatment.

In practice, a reasonable course of action would start with explaining to the patient why you think it is necessary that the health-care team knows about his HIV status. The patient should also be informed that all health-care staff (and students) are under a duty of confidentiality, and in particular, a GP is not well placed to manage the patient's condition unless she is informed about the patient's HIV status. However, with regards to informing a GP, if the patient continues to refuse a disclosure, his wishes in general ought to be respected. Rarely, for example if the patient is violent or severely mentally disturbed,

disclosure to the GP without consent may be appropriate.

What then of disclosing information to the patient's partner? One way of thinking about what to do is to try and weigh up relative benefits and harms caused by disclosure and by non-disclosure. The harm of disclosure is the breach of confidentiality and resultant loss of privacy of the patient. The benefits are the potential avoidance of a serious life-threatening risk to the patient's partner. It seems reasonably uncontroversial that preventing a loss of life is better than preventing a loss of privacy. Some people have argued that doctors have a duty of care only toward patients (not their partners) and as such do not need to look out for the interests of such individuals. This view is not generally accepted.

The GMC advises that you should disclose information in order to protect a person from risk of death or serious harm. However, you must not disclose information to relatives or others who have not been, and are not, at risk of infection. The approach of the courts has been to consider the public interest in maintaining confidentiality (confidentiality encourages patients to seek treatment) against the public interest in disclosure (protection of people at risk).

Confidentiality and HIV

- In general, difficulties that arise around the issue of confidentiality and HIV can be addressed by open and honest discussion with the patient.
- If after counselling, a patient refuses that their GP be informed about their HIV status, then this wish should be respected – unless the doctor is judged to be at risk of infection.
- If after counselling, a patient refuses to inform their partner (who may have been, or is continuing to be exposed to infection), it is not improper to inform the partner against the wishes of the patient. However, the patient must be told of the intention to inform.

Common problems in medical practice

Public expectations of the medical profession have noticeably changed since the advent of the NHS. The attitude of 'doctor knows best' has waned: a sociological change mirrored in ethics by a move from paternalism to the autonomy-based approaches of today. In 1991, the Patient's Charter set out the standards that patients had a right to expect from the NHS. These were presented as ten patient's rights, which included minimum waiting times, levels of information to be provided, the right to treatment on the basis of need rather than ability to pay and so on. The Patient's Charter has subsequently been updated. Further changes have been imposed upon hospitals; over 100 targets (on cleanliness, waiting times, and numbers of procedures and so on) are imposed by central government.

These changes, along with an increasingly litigious and rights-conscious society, have contributed to a more consumerist approach to patients. Indeed, the Patient's Charter refers to patients as 'care consumers'. Much debate has focused on whether the strengthening of patients' rights has helped or hindered the provision of care based on clinical need. It has undoubtedly, however, led to an increased scrutiny of how the medical profession and the provision of care are regulated.

Professional regulation

The Royal College of Physicians came into being in the 16th century. They were the first body to be responsible for examinations and registration of doctors. The British Medical Association (BMA) was established in 1832. The BMA's main function is to protect the interests of its members; it is a trade union for doctors. However, it was the BMA that lobbied for the creation of the GMC. This was established by an Act of Parliament (the Medical Registration Act 1858). The GMC is the governing body of the medical profession. The functions of the GMC are broadly:

- To set professional standards.
- To ensure that those allowed to practise medicine (registered medical practitioners) are fit to do so.
- A supervision of standards of education – the GMC sets out a syllabus for medical schools to follow.
- The enforcement of professional discipline – the ultimate sanction is to 'strike a doctor off the register' either temporarily or permanently.

The GMC sets out guidelines called *Duties of a Doctor* on what it deems to be good practice (Fig. 2.3). These guidelines are important because they represent the opinion of a respected body of medical professionals. For this reason the guidelines are often relied upon in court, and a doctor who has not followed guidelines will be expected to justify why he hasn't.

The NHS complaints procedure

The current NHS complaints procedure was instituted in 1996 by the NHS Executive. It was titled: *'Complaints, Listening . . . Acting . . . Improving: Guidance on Implementation of the NHS Complaints Procedure'*. The aims of this complaints procedure are to provide a simple, responsive way of tackling complaints, with the goal of improving the level of service provided by the NHS. In essence it proposes three tiers of response to complaints. The complaints procedure is an alternative to legal action. If a patient expresses the desire to take a health authority to court, the complaints procedure is stopped.

Most complaints should be dealt with at a local level. This would involve the person about whom the complaint was made responding either in writing or in person to the complainant. Hospital trusts provide a lay conciliator to facilitate such meetings. The idea is that with honest and open communication, the complainant and the person complained about can see each other's points of view, and resolution to the satisfaction of both parties can be achieved.

If a complainant is not satisfied by attempts at local resolution, he/she can request an independent review of the complaint. All Trusts will have a complaints convenor who will decide whether to set up an independent review panel or return the complaint to the local level. There is no automatic right to independent review, and the complainant must state a case for why local resolution has been unsatisfactory.

An independent review panel consists of three lay members advised by clinical specialists. The function of the panel is to investigate the complaint and make a report setting out its conclusions, with appropriate comments and suggestions. It cannot suggest that any person should be subject to disciplinary action or referred to any of the professional regulatory bodies.

The report is sent to the chief executive of the trust, who must then write to the complainant informing them of any action that is being taken as a result of the panel's deliberations and the right of the

---

The GMC's *Duties of a Doctor*

The GMC produces a number of booklets including the following:

Good Medical Practice

This starts with the principle that:

> All patients are entitled to good standards of practice and care from their doctors. Essential elements of this are professional competence; good relationships with patients and colleagues; and observance of professional ethical obligations

It also covers what good standards of practice and care entail, as well as recommendations about how to make medical decisions, how to keep up to date, maintaining trust with patients and colleagues, how to deal with complaints, professional probity and what to do if doctors believe their own health is putting patients at risk

---

Seeking Patients' Consent: the Ethical Considerations

This starts with:

> Successful relationships between doctors and patients depend on trust. To establish that trust you must respect patients' autonomy – their right to decide whether or not to undergo any medical intervention even where a refusal may result in harm to themselves or in their own death

It outlines the necessity of providing sufficient information, responding to questions, where information can be withheld and how to present information to patients

---

Conficentiality: Protecting and Providing Information

This starts with:

> Patients have a right to expect that information about them will be held in confidence by their doctors

Conficentiality is discussed earlier on in this chapter

Serious Communicable Diseases
This starts with the reminder that:

> All patients are entitled to good standards of practice and care from their doctors, regardless of the nature of their disease or condition

The booklet gives guidance on how to obtain consent to testing for diseases such as HIV, tuberculosis and hepatitis B and C. It also deals with how to respond to needlestick injuries, research, and disclosure to others

---

Available as booklets from the GMC or online at *www.gmc-uk.org*

Other booklets cover research, withholding and withdrawing life-prolonging treatments, management in health care and the new doctor.

Fig. 2.3 The GMC's *Duties of a Doctor*.

complainant to take their grievance to the ombudsman if they remain dissatisfied. It is up to the chief executive to decide whether or not to refer the cases to a professional body (e.g. the GMC) or initiate their own disciplinary procedures.

The ombudsman (or health service commissioner) is a civil servant, independent of the NHS, who is responsible for reporting to parliament about the running of the NHS. It is up to the ombudsman whether or not to further investigate any complaints. It is within his power to ask health-care professionals involved in complaints to appear before a parliamentary select committee in order to give their account of the subject of the complaint. This complaints procedure provides no avenue for the complainant to be compensated. In order to do this the complainant needs to use the civil justice system, as outlined in Chapter 1.

Dealing with uncertainty and conflict

Medicine has been described as the least accurate of the sciences. The inaccuracy means that sometimes

NHS complaints procedure
Level 1 – Local resolution
Level 2 – Independent review
Level 3 – Ombudsman

treatment is not successful or outcomes are less than hoped for by doctors and patients. Evidence-based medicine (EBM) is the approved approach to dealing with those questions where uncertainty exists. This is dealt with in Chapter 9.

However, what should the doctor 'at the coalface' do when unsure of the way forward? One response has been to practise what has become known as 'defensive medicine'. This is to do the investigations and treatment that will ensure the least chance of being sued, rather than ensuring the best outcome for the patient.

Clinical mistakes and whistle-blowing

Mistakes happen in all workplaces; however, given that medicine does literally deal with matters of life and death, the results of mistakes may be considerably more grave than those made in other walks of life. The Bristol Royal Infirmary Inquiry addressed the question of how to learn from mistakes. This inquiry identified a 'culture of blame and stigma' within the NHS. How then should students and doctors react when they realize they have made a mistake? How should they react if they become aware that one of their colleagues is making mistakes?

If you make a mistake, a reasonable course of action may be to:

- Inform a senior colleague.
- Apologize to the patient and explain why the mistake was made – also explain the consequences of the mistake. The patient may wish to speak to a more senior doctor, and depending on the gravity of the mistake this may be appropriate.
- Inform the patient of the mistake and what steps are being taken to rectify it.
- It is difficult to ethically justify *not* telling the patient that a mistake has been made.

If you believe that a colleague is unfit to practise medicine you could:

- Consider whether or not patients are at risk – your primary concern is the safety of patients.
- If you feel able to, you could approach your colleague directly and voice your concerns. You may be able to reach an agreement whereby your colleague takes time off work and seeks professional help.
- If you are uncomfortable approaching your colleague directly, or your colleague denies there is

a problem, you should voice your concerns to an appropriate person from the employing authority, for example the medical director, or your colleague's educational supervisor. If the concern is about a medical problem such as drug/alcohol addiction, psychiatric illness or a serious infectious disease, you may wish to speak to a consultant occupational doctor (see below).

- You may wish to discuss your options with your defence organization or the GMC.

The Public Interest Disclosure Act 1998, which is sometimes called the 'Whistle-Blowing Act', is designed to protect from victimization and dismissal those employees who report their concerns about the performance of colleagues (to the appropriate authorities).

Occupational health

What then are the sorts of problems that would lead to health-care professionals requiring help from an occupational-health department? The GMC is not completely specific, rather it talks about any condition that leads to a colleague 'placing patients at risk as a result of illness or another medical condition'. One envisages that this could include the following:

- Serious communicable diseases: particularly HIV, tuberculosis, hepatitis B and C. The GMC recommends that if you believe a medical colleague has a serious communicable disease and is continuing to practise *in a way which places patients at risk*, you must inform an appropriate person in the health-care worker's employing authority, such as an occupational health physician. Of course, doctors with disease are allowed to continue to practise; however, they may be restricted in the invasive procedures they perform.
- Psychiatric disorders, including depression (that hinders the ability of the doctor to properly care for her patients), personality disorders and psychotic disorders.
- Alcohol and drug addiction.

 It is important to determine whether or not patients are at risk because of the behaviour or illness of the health professional.

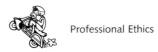

Ethics in medical research

A brief history of guidelines and abuse in medical research
~425 BC
The Hippocratic Oath, whilst making no mention of research, does have a clause advocating doing only that which benefits patients: 'Into whatever houses I enter, I will go into them for the benefit of the sick, and will abstain from every voluntary act of mischief and corruption.'

1900
Ironically, one of the first codes of conduct was a directive from the Prussian Minister of Religious, Educational and Medical Affairs. According to this directive medical experimentation could be conducted only on competent adults who had consented after a proper explanation of the adverse consequences that might result. This was in force during the Third Reich, but flouted.

1932–70
The US Public Health Service undertook an experiment to study the progression of syphilis. This took place in Tuskegee where up to 400 black men with syphilis were studied. They were denied effective treatment (penicillin) even after it became available.

1940–45
'Medical experiments' were carried out in Nazi Germany under the direction of Dr Josef Mengele. Human subjects were treated like, or indeed worse than, animals in medical research.

1947
World Medical Association (WMA) issued the *Declaration of Geneva* – basically an updated version of the Hippocratic Oath. This includes the phrase: *'The health of my patient will be my first consideration.'*

1949
The Nuremburg Court specified ten points – known as the '*Nuremburg Code*' – as a result of the case *United States v. Brandt*. (Brandt was Hitler's personal physician – although the case also heard 19 other Third Reich doctors and three biomedical scientists; and the trial was conducted under US military patronage.) The ten points included:

1. An *absolute* need for *voluntary* consent.
2. A justification in terms of potential 'fruitful results'.
3. Proper design and previous animal experiments.
4. The avoidance of 'unnecessary physical and mental suffering and injury'.
5. The conduct of the experiment by 'scientifically qualified persons'.
6. The termination of the experiment if it becomes clear that harm will result or if the human subject wishes to bring it to an end.

1954
WMA adopted a Code for Research and Experimentation that allowed proxy consent; effectively a weakening of the position of the Nuremburg Code.

1964
Declaration of Helsinki (updated 1975, 1983, 1989, 1996, and 2000) allowed for some experimentation on human subjects including the very young, the unconscious, and those who lack legal capacity such as the mentally ill. More popular with the medical profession as the Nuremburg Code is more restrictive.

1968
Informal research ethics committees established in the UK after a report by the Royal College of Physicians; these are non-statutory bodies composed of members drawn predominantly from the health professions (although there are some lay members) to consider proposals for clinical trials.

1984 and 1990
Principal guidelines covering research in UK issued by the Royal College of Physicians require that experimentation be subject to ethical review prior to being carried out. The guidelines make a number of recommendations about the review process:

> Where the administration of effective treatment is important for the future well-being of the patient, it is ethical for a controlled trial to be undertaken only if, at the outset, the investigator does not know whether the trial treatment is more effective or less effective than the standard treatment with which it is to be compared (or than no treatment at all in the case of a placebo controlled study)' – *Author's note: this is the position of equipoise* (see below).

7.99

28

Withholding effective treatment for a short time . . . can sometimes be acceptable . . . patient consent is necessary and the patient may agree that he need not know precisely when this will take place

7.100

. . . If a patient expresses a strong preference for a particular treatment, he is probably ineligible as a participant

7.103

. . . randomization of treatment without the consent of the patient is unethical

7.105

1991
Department of Health issues guidelines (HSG(91)5) to local research ethics committees.

1997
Department of Health issues guidelines (HSG(97)23) to establish multi-centre research ethics committees.

2000
Declaration of Helsinki revised.

2001
Governance arrangements for NHS research ethics committees. This document provided a framework for the process of review of the ethics of all proposals for research in the NHS and social care.

2001
International Conference on Harmonization – Guidelines for Good Clinical Practice. This sets out an international ethical and scientific standard for research on human subjects. It is consistent with the principles of the Declaration of Helsinki and it aims to provide a unified standard for the European Union, Japan and the USA.

2001
EU Directive 2001/20/EC published.
This directive governs research on human subjects in the EU.

The ethical issues at stake in medical research
Given the starting point that there isn't complete knowledge about how diseases progress and how best to treat them, medical research of some sort is necessary. The benefits of research include reducing future human suffering and contributing to the sum of human knowledge. However, previous abuses, under the auspices of medical research, require us to remain vigilant in order that the rights of the individual are not ignored. Thus, there exists a tension between reducing future suffering and the rights of the individual.

Medical research in the UK is subject to ethical review by a research ethics committee. In 1991, The Department of Health required that every health district set up a local research ethics committee to scrutinize the ethical justification for local medical research. These committees require a multi-disciplinary approach and commonly consist of lay members, clinicians, and often a philosopher/theologian and/or a statistician/scientist. What then do these committees look for in research proposals? How do they weigh potential public benefit against potential harm to individuals?

1. *The position of equipoise*: In order to carry out medical research, you must be in a position of equipoise – this means that it isn't *known* whether the experimental treatment is any more effective than current treatments. You should have reason to believe that it is, for example it has been demonstrated to be more effective in animal studies, but have no actual evidence. This means there is a responsibility to ensure that the research proposed hasn't already been carried out.
2. *A clear purpose*: You must establish a need for doing the proposed experiment – it is important not only that there is a position of equipoise before the experiment, but that when the experiment is completed, the results will in some way be important. If the experiment is not scientifically valid, then it is unlikely that it will be ethically justifiable.
3. *The principle of least harm*: You should ensure that the experiment's design allows only the minimal amount of harm to befall the individual. This usually means that experiments should compare a new treatment against the current standard treatment, rather than against a placebo. You must demonstrate that the potential benefits are greater than the potential risks of the treatment.
4. *Consent*: Before commencing research, the participants should give their fully informed consent to take part. You must inform patients of the potential risks and benefits, and, if appropriate, whether or not they will randomly

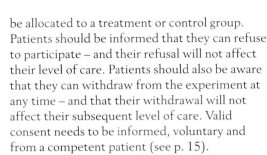

be allocated to a treatment or control group. Patients should be informed that they can refuse to participate – and their refusal will not affect their level of care. Patients should also be aware that they can withdraw from the experiment at any time – and that their withdrawal will not affect their subsequent level of care. Valid consent needs to be informed, voluntary and from a competent patient (see p. 15).

5. *The difference between therapeutic and non-therapeutic research*: Therapeutic research involves giving patients an experimental treatment in order to see how effective it is. Non-therapeutic research involves giving a treatment to healthy individuals. That is, therapeutic research has potential benefits for the patient, whereas non-therapeutic research does not. Many people believe that non-therapeutic research should involve lower levels of risk – because there is little area for benefit. This distinction has been dropped from the 2000 Helsinki Revision, but still has legal force with respect to children and those decisions to include individuals in a trial in their *best interests*.

The philosophical approach one uses can determine whether or not certain risks are acceptable (Figs 2.4 & 2.5).

Research on vulnerable groups

In ethical terms, a vulnerable group is any group that lacks the ability to make informed choices about themselves. Thus, vulnerable individuals include children, the incapacitated, the mentally ill and groups that may be easily exploited (for example prisoners or those in the third world).

Research in children

The basic problem posed by children is that they are not always able to give valid consent. They may be competent to make some decisions, but not others (p. 49). Children over 16 are able to consent to medical treatment and possibly therapeutic research. Children under 16 *may* be sufficiently competent to give such consent as well. However, if a child is incompetent, consent to participate in research should be obtained from an individual with parental responsibility. Furthermore, the risks of the research must be sufficiently low to say that participating in the research is still in the best interests of the child. Whether or not a child can take part in non-therapeutic research is contentious. However, if the research involves something relatively low-risk, for example taking a blood sample, then it may be ethically defensible to allow such research (assuming the other criteria above were met). If at all possible, it would be better to seek the child's assent to the procedure, even if fully informed consent cannot be obtained.

Research in incapacitated adults and adults with mental disabilities

Research in this group has some parallels with that in children, but unlike the situation with children, in UK law, no-one can consent on behalf of adults. All treatment, which includes being entered for a trial, is

A comparison of three different ethical approaches to research	High-risk research where participants are *not* fully informed	High-risk research where participants *are* fully informed	Low-risk research where participants are *not* fully informed	Low-risk research where participants *are* fully informed	Poor-quality research: *low risks* but patients *are* fully informed
Libertarian (rights based)	No	Yes	No	Yes	Yes
Paternalistic (duty based)	No	No	Yes	Yes	?No
Utilitarian (consequentialist)	?No	Yes	Yes	Yes	No

Fig. 2.4 A comparison of three different ethical approaches to research.

Source: adapted from Hope T, Salvulescu J, Hendrick J 2003 *Medical Ethics and Law: the core curriculum.* Edinburgh: Churchill Livingstone

Fig. 2.5 Phases of clinical trials.

Phases of clinical trials

Phase One:

Study of pharmacokinetics and pharmacodynamics
Aim to confirm safe dosages for patients
Use *healthy* volunteers
Placebo comparisons common
Small numbers of participants (order of tens)

Phase Two:

Aim to demonstrate efficacy of new agent
Use *real patients* with the disease for which the new agent is intended
Comparison with established agent or placebo
Larger numbers of participants (order of hundreds)

Phase Three:

Aim to demonstrate superiority of new agent
Use *real patients* often in *double blind* trials
Comparison between new agent, existing therapy and if possible placebo
Very large numbers of participants (order of thousands)
Results used as basis for request for licensing

Phase Four:

Conducted after agent is licensed
Aim to determine long-term efficacy and safety
Way of refining optimal doses and identifying categories of patients who do not respond to treatment
Variable number of participants

Source: adapted from Schwartz L, Preece PE, Hendry RA 2002 Medical Ethics: A case-based approach. Edinburgh: Saunders, p. 193

made on the basis of the patient's best interests. However, it is hard to justify proceeding with experimental treatment on incapacitated adults (for example stroke victims) without consulting relatives first, simply because this shows a willingness to communicate and a desire to find out what the patient's wishes would have been if they were able to express them.

Animal research

The ethics of animal research are not clear cut. There exists a range of animals used in research and it is not obvious that standards appropriate for treating mice are necessarily the same as the standards we think ought to exist for experiments on primates. Furthermore, there exist good and bad experiments; some with the potential to provide significant benefits to mankind and some that won't. As a result, it tends to be a bit simplistic to either say that animal experiments should be allowed or that they shouldn't. Rather more

debate is centred on what sort of potential benefit justifies experimenting on animals.

A useful list of points to consider when deciding whether a particular experiment justifies the use of animals might be as follows:

1. Is the experiment well designed, and will it produce significant results?
2. Could the experiment be done without using laboratory animals?
3. Will animal suffering be maximally alleviated, for example if the experiment involves new surgical techniques, will the animals used be given anaesthetic and analgesic agents as well as agents for muscle paralysis?
4. When using primates for research, consider the following question 'Is this the sort of research we would be happy doing to humans with a mental capacity that is equivalent to that of the animals being used? If not, why are we happy to do it on primates but not the mentally ill?'

A Select Committee on Animals in Scientific Procedures reported in 2002 that:

- It is morally acceptable for human beings to use other animals for research, but it is morally wrong to cause them unnecessary or avoidable suffering.
- There is a continued need for animal experiments both in applied research and in research aimed purely at extending knowledge.
- There is scope for the pursuit of the three Rs of animal research.

The three Rs of animal research:
Replacement of conscious, living animals by non-sentient alternatives
Reduction in the number of animals needed to obtain information of a given amount and precision
Refinement of procedures so as to produce the minimal amount or severity of suffering experienced by those animals which have to be used.

Ethics in resource allocation

Resource allocation within the NHS is one of the most intractable ethical problems. No health service in the world is able to provide the best available treatment for every single patient that could benefit from it. The NHS, in attempting to provide a 'cradle to the grave' service, largely without a private sector input, is more stretched than most.

Broadly speaking there are two levels of resource allocation:

1. Micro-allocation: decisions about treatment between patients.
2. Macro-allocation: decisions over the share of a society's total resources which are devoted to health, and the division of the health-care budget between possible uses (Harris 2001).

Doctors tend to be concerned with decisions of micro-allocation, i.e. deciding which patients get which treatments. Health Authorities and the Government make decisions regarding macro-allocation.

Why is resource allocation necessary?

The usual answer to this question is that resources (money, doctors and other health professionals, equipment and so on) are not infinite, thus scarcity becomes inevitable. With scarcity comes a need to decide who receives treatment and who does not.

Remember: whilst resources are not infinite, they are not finite either – they are indefinite. Any budget can be traded off other budgets – priorities can be reassessed – so if this year the budget for the NHS is £130 billion, it could be increased next year if people are happy to pay higher rates of tax. Demand for a service is not inevitably infinite – rather 'the amount demanded of a free service is determined at the point where customers see no additional benefits to be gained from additional recourse to the service in question'. This can be at quite modest levels (Harris 2001).

Having said this, it is generally accepted that some decisions have to be made with regard to the allocation of resources. If this is the case, what are the grounds upon which rationing decisions could be made? The following are some suggestions regarding the grounds upon which we could choose between claimants:

- Increase in *quantity* of life as a result of treatment.
- Increase in *quality* of life as a result of treatment.
- *Prognosis* – treat those with the best *chance* of a successful outcome.
- Past *contribution* or future (expected) *contribution* to society – who has paid the most taxes? Or will do in the future?
- *Personal responsibility* – should smokers and alcoholics have equal access to health care as people without such harmful habits? What about skiers and people injured whilst quad biking? What about risky professions, such as firemen?
- *Moral character* and fault – de-prioritize treatment for those seen to be at fault, such as drunken drivers in accidents?
- *Triage* – immediate treatment will help? Can wait but need treatment? No point treating?

In the rest of this section a number of alternative theoretical foundations for deciding how to allocate scarce resources will be analysed.

Quality adjusted life years

The quality adjusted life years (QALY) theory is an approach to cost-effectiveness and is a *utilitarian* theory (see also p. 78). It attempts to bring two

considerations into a single framework when assessing the cost-effectiveness of health-care interventions:
1. Quality of life
and
2. Quantity of life.

These two criteria are used because both are thought to be central to the purpose of health care. Medicine is not seen simply as a method of saving lives (increasing *life years*); part of its role is to alleviate suffering, that is improve *quality*. QALYs combine both criteria in a single measurement.

This theory was developed by Williams, who wrote:

> The essence of a QALY is that it takes a year of health life expectancy to be worth 1, but regards a year of unhealthy life expectancy as worth less than 1. Its precise value is lower the worse the quality of life of the unhealthy person (which is what the 'quality adjusted' bit is all about).
>
> (Williams 1985)

This theory allows health-care interventions to be scored according to how many QALYs they result in. When this is considered along with the cost of an intervention, health interventions can be considered in terms of *cost per QALY*. This allows cost-effective analysis to take place. Without such a system, it can be hard to compare widely divergent medical treatments.

QALYs allow two sorts of decisions to be made when choosing health care. These are:
1. To determine which therapy is given to an individual patient: this is effectively a decision made according to the rules of evidence-based medicine.
2. To determine which patients receive treatment at all: a cost-effective analysis.

Like utilitarianism, QALYs are popular because they tap into two main moral intuitions. First, that we *ought* to promote *well-being* as measured: the 'quality' part, and, second, that we *ought* to *maximize* the amount of well-being: the 'quantity'.

Objections to quality adjusted life years
Two of the major problems with QALYs are:
1. QALYs are arguably *unjust*.
2. QALYs are arguably *difficult to calculate practically*.

The argument from justice claims that QALYs are systematically biased against certain sections of the population and that this means they are an unfair basis upon which to allocate resources. Those groups which aren't favoured by the QALY system include the disabled, the chronically ill and the elderly. This bias is illustrated by considering the following case.

Imagine Tom, Dick and Harry are in a car crash. Tom is 20 years old with no previous disabilities. Dick is also 20 years old and is blind. Harry is 40 and was previously well. The car crash results in all three sustaining similar injuries, for example a fractured pelvis. They all arrive at A&E at the same time, but the hospital has enough resources (for example orthopaedic surgeons or blood) for only one patient.

Assuming that all three patients could be returned to the same level of health they had before the accident, the QALY system would oblige the hospital to treat Tom over the other two. The reasons for this are that Tom will live longer than Harry (assuming both have an average life-span), therefore, even though both can be returned to perfect health, treating Tom will lead to a greater number of QALYs being accrued. (Assuming the average life expectancy to be 75, treating Tom will lead to 55 QALYs versus 35 QALYs for Harry.) Whilst many people think that we should treat children in preference to the very old, it becomes less clear whether we should treat 20 year olds instead of 40 year olds, or 30 year olds instead of 35 year olds.

Tom will also be treated in preference to Dick, although both have the same life expectancy. Because Dick already has a disability, treating his fractured pelvis will not restore him to *perfect* health. Each year of life after treatment will be worth less than 1 on the QALY scale – so his total expected QALY score will be less than 55. John Harris has called this problem 'double jeopardy' (Harris 1995); not only does Dick have the misfortune to be blind, but this disability can also, under the QALY system, adversely affect the priority assigned to him in receiving treatment for an unrelated injury.

The problem of *calculating* QALYs is a more practical difficulty. For example, how can we compare the quality of life of being blind as against that of being paralysed? The answer tends to depend both on how the question is asked and which groups of individuals answer the question. Disabled groups tend to rate their quality of life much higher than do non-disabled groups.

Rawls' theory of justice
John Rawls utilizes a hypothetical device he calls the '*veil of ignorance*' – this is part of an explanatory model to explain an ideal social contract – for Rawls

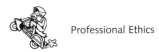

this is the type of contract it would be rational to choose if we had been given the chance. Unlike the QALY theory, the supreme goal in Rawls' theory of justice is not maximization of welfare as such, but treating those who have the greatest need for treatment. This theory emphasizes fairness rather than absolute welfare.

Rawls supposes:
• Humans are rational.

and

• Humans are self-interested.

Thus, in order to further fairness (justice), steps must be taken to avoid selfish interest in the original position (from which the social contract is made) as follows:

1. If people are self-interested, they will seek advantages at the expense of others whenever they can.

BUT

2. If people did not know how to advantage themselves, they would not 'rationally' try to advantage themselves.

HENCE

3. The veil of ignorance disguises salient information that they could use to advantage themselves.

THEREFORE

4. If we can suppose what the social contract would have been, had it been designed from behind a veil of ignorance, it would be just (i.e. fair).

AND

5. If we could be sure of this, it would also be fair to hold people to this in the real world.

Working under this model, Rawls produced two important principles:

1. People would choose to have an equal right to the most extensive basic liberties compatible with everyone having those liberties: that is, there would be MAXIMUM FREEDOM.

2. Because people are rationally self-interested, they will adopt a MAXIMIN POLICY (i.e. a worst-case scenario). As people don't know where they will be in society, they will accept the prudence of making the situation of those on the

• Why is telling the truth important?
• Name a principle that would lead to truth-telling and one that would lead to non-disclosure of information.
• What legal cases have set precedents in the disclosure of risk?
• Who decides what constitutes a *real* risk?
• What is paternalism? What are three arguments for it and three against it?
• What are the problems with asserting there is a '*right not to know*' information?
• What is necessary for *informed consent*?
• What is the *Re C Test* used for?
• What is the *Bolam Test* used for?
• How should doctors act in cases where the patient is incompetent?
• When can confidential information be disclosed?
• Which statutes grant patients access to their health records?
• What is the role of the General Medical Council?
• Outline five ethical issues at stake in medical research.
• What is the difference between micro-allocation and macro-allocation?
• Outline three problems with QALYs.
• What is the *veil of ignorance*?

lowest rung as good as possible (MAXImum welfare for the MINimally well off).

References
Gert B, Culver C 1979 The justification of paternalism. Ethics 2(199–210): 204
Harris J 1995 Double jeopardy and the veil of ignorance – a reply. Journal of Medical Ethics 21: 151–7
Harris J 2001 Micro-allocation: deciding between patients. In: Singer PA (ed.) Companion to Bioethics. Oxford: Blackwell Publishers
Häyry H 1998 Paternalism. In: Chadwick R (ed.) Encyclopedia of Applied Ethics, Vol. 3. London: Academic Press
Williams A 1985 The value of QALYs. Health and Social Service Journal (Centre 8 Supplement) pp. 3–5

Further reading
General Medical Council 2000 Confidentiality: Protecting and Providing Information. London: General Medical Council
Rawls J 1972 A Theory of Justice. Oxford: Oxford University Press
Singer PA (ed.) 2001 Companion to Bioethics. Oxford: Blackwell Publishers

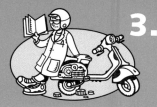

3. Applied Ethics

Reproduction and genetics

The human embryo

Human reproduction is a fertile ground for ethical dilemmas. The reason for this is that unlike the rest of medicine, health-care professionals see themselves as responsible for two entities – the patient *and* the unborn child. Ethical problems can be seen to arise where there is conflict between the best interests of the mother and those of the embryo, fetus or potential child. The clearest example of this conflict is perhaps apparent in the ethics of abortion. However, a common thread of argument may run through a number of the issues in reproductive ethics. One's ethical stance on abortion, *in vitro fertilization* (IVF), cloning and genetic screening may largely be determined by one's view on the moral status of the embryo or fetus. The legal status of the fetus is clear: it has no legal rights. However, how should we determine the *moral* value of the embryo? A number of views, and objections, are presented below.

The embryo is morally valuable because it is a human organism

This view holds that the value of the embryo is situated in the fact that it is *human* and as such deserves moral recognition. This view would hold that if it is morally wrong to kill an adult, it would have been equally wrong to kill that same person when she was a child, fetus or embryo because all of these entities are part of a continuous individual identity that can be traced back to conception.

But:

- Is killing a zygote, or a primitive embryo, really as morally bad as killing a child? One way of thinking about this is to imagine a scenario where you are able to save either an embryo (in a test tube) or a five-year-old child from a fire in a laboratory. Would you be morally justified in saving the embryo? If not, why not?
- Why are human embryos more important than other embryos? What characteristics do early human embryos (for example at the 8- or 16-cell stage) have that distinguish them from other

mammalian embryos, apart from potential to develop into humans?

The embryo is morally valuable because it is a potential human being

This view accepts that the embryo is not morally valuable in and of itself. However, because it can potentially develop into a human child, it deserves moral concern. Killing an embryo is wrong because it deprives the child that could have potentially lived its existence. This view also generally holds that moral concern starts at conception.

But:

- If it is potentiality that is important, are gametes deserving of moral concern as well? For example, a couple that uses contraception is effectively preventing a number of potential children being realized.

The embryo/fetus is morally valuable if it is a 'person'

This view holds that there is some characteristic or characteristics that morally valuable entities have. Such entities may be referred to as 'persons'. Different people hold different characteristics to confer moral status. However, common characteristics of personhood include: consciousness (or perhaps *self-consciousness*), sentience, rationality, the ability to form future plans and the capacity to value one's own life. A religious view may hold that embryos are not persons until the soul enters the body – that is until ensoulment. This may be at conception or at a later stage.

Remember that in this context 'being a *person*' is not the same as 'being a *human being*'. Some humans may not qualify as persons, and some non-humans may qualify as persons!

But:

- Some of these characteristics will confer the status of personhood on embryos beyond a certain stage of development; for example after 24 weeks a fetus can probably feel pain, so would qualify as a person if sentience was the criterion being used. However, others, like self-consciousness or the capacity to value one's own life, require a far greater degree of development, and indeed may exclude newborns and infants from 'personhood'.

- Some characteristics may also exclude individuals with severe learning difficulties, leaving some question as to how these individuals are to be treated.
- Some characteristics may include other animals; we have no reason to doubt that all other mammals are able to feel pain in a similar way to humans, and some higher primates may be self-conscious.

The embryo is morally valuable because it is valued by others

This view holds that embryos are morally valuable because they are the objects of moral concern to others. This means that the value of the embryo is not *intrinsic*, but is conferred by others. Thus the wrong in killing an embryo, fetus or even an infant is not the wrong done to that entity, but is wrong because there exist individuals (for example the parents) who care for it, and do not wish it to be harmed. There also exists a broader concern that the killing of such entities would diminish the concern for older children, and human life in general.

But:

- Does this mean it would be acceptable to kill newborns if no-one around them cared? Such a thought does not readily sit with many who think that infants are important in themselves.

The moral value of the embryo increases as it continues to develop

This viewpoint accepts that the moral value of the zygote is less than that of the embryo, which in turn is less than that of the newborn. This view avoids the arbitrary nature of the first two, which hold that moral value crystallizes at conception. Its strength is that it doesn't specify a particular stage of development that is of over-riding importance. This, however, can also be seen as a weakness, in that it doesn't provide practical guidance on whether abortion at 12 weeks, 24 weeks or term is morally acceptable.

Abortion

The abortion debate is perhaps one of the longest-running ethical debates. In ancient Greek and Roman times both abortion and infanticide were practised. The fetus and infant were seen to be products of the mother and as such 'owned' by the husband who was free to dispose of the infant in anyway he saw fit. In general, Christianity forbade abortion, although arguments were put forward between the 15th and 18th centuries that claimed abortions prior to the mother feeling the fetus move (a time known as the 'quickening') were permissible on the grounds that ensoulment was yet to happen. In the 18th and 19th centuries 'medical opinion' accepted 'preformism' – the idea that spermatozoa contained a fully formed, miniature, human being (known as a *homunculus*) and that the uterus simply provided a fertile environment for a diminutive person to grow. Such a view was used to bolster anti-abortion arguments. It wasn't until the first quarter of the 20th century that a good understanding of the science of reproduction was obtained. However, abortion remained illegal in most Western countries until the 1960s.

Abortion legislation

There are two important statutes to consider in the law on abortion:

1. Offences Against the Person Act 1861, ss. 58–59: these sections make illegal:
   a. the self-induction of miscarriage
   b. a second person helping a woman to procure an abortion
   c. the supply or procurement of an abortifacient.
2. Abortion Act 1967, amended 1990.

The Abortion Act 1967 was designed to tackle two main problems. The first was that of back-street abortions, which were leading to significant injury in women. The second was the result of a common-law decision that suggested that abortions were acceptable if the doctor believed a continuation of the pregnancy would 'make the woman a physical or mental wreck'. This decision led to the problem of doctors thinking they were carrying out abortions in good faith, but at the same time running the risk of facing criminal charges.

Figure 3.1 shows an important section of the Abortion Act 1967 (as amended 1990). It is also worth noting the following points:

1. In general the opinion of two doctors is needed – this, however, is not the case in an emergency.
2. Ss.1(1a) allows an abortion to be carried out before the 24th week of pregnancy for a wide variety of reasons, including preventing harm to a woman's existing children. This clause is sometimes referred to as the 'statistical clause', as statistically *any* normal pregnancy carries more risk than a standard early termination, thus according to some it effectively allows any abortion to fulfil the criteria

The Abortion Act 1967 ss. 1 (1–2)

Fig. 3.1 The Abortion Act 1967 ss. 1 (1–2).

1. Subject to the provisions of this section, a person shall not be guilty of an offence under the law relating to abortion when a pregnancy is terminated by a registered medical practitioner if two registered medical practitioners are of the opinion, formed in good faith:

a. that the pregnancy has not exceeded its 24th week and that the continuance of the pregnancy would involve risk, greater than if the pregnancy were terminated, of injury to the physical or mental health of the pregnant woman or any existing children of her family

or

b. that the termination is necessary to prevent grave permanent injury to the physical or mental health of the pregnant woman

or

c. that the continuance of the pregnancy would involve risk to the life of the pregnant woman, greater than if the pregnancy were terminated

or

d. that there is substantial risk that if the child were born, it would suffer from such physical or mental abnormalities as to be seriously handicapped

2. In determining whether the continuance of a pregnancy would involve such risk of injury to health as is mentioned in paragraph (a) or (b) of subsection (1) of this section, account may be taken of the pregnant woman's actual or reasonably foreseeable environment

of the Act. Most abortions take place under this section.

3. The Abortion Act does not give women the *right* to demand an abortion. The power to decide whether a woman qualifies for an abortion lies with the medical practitioner. The woman's *consent* is necessary and she can of course *refuse* to have an abortion even if it is thought necessary to save her own life.

4. If the woman is unable to give consent, then an abortion can still be carried out if it is in the woman's *best interests* and in accordance with good medical practice.

5. After the 24th week of pregnancy, risk to the life of the woman, the prevention of serious disability, or fetal disability (most common) is required for an abortion to be carried out.

6. The fetus does *not* have any legal rights.

7. The father of the fetus has no legal right to prevent the woman from having an abortion.

8. The Abortion Act gives doctors the right to make a 'conscientious objection' to participating 'in any treatment authorized by [the] Act' except in an emergency. However, the doctor must not prevent the woman from obtaining access to abortion services. For example, if a patient sees her GP and requests an abortion, the GP must refer her if she meets the criteria of the Abortion

Act, even if he personally thinks abortion is morally wrong.

9. If in a late abortion the fetus is born alive, then doctors have a legal obligation to try and save it. This is because the killing of a fetus once it is outside the uterus falls under the definition of homicide.

The ethical arguments for and against abortion

The ethical argument tends to be framed by opposing positions:

- The '*pro-life*' position: the extreme version of this view holds that all human life is sacrosanct and, therefore, abortion is the moral equivalent of homicide. Arguments are in general made either from the position that all human organisms are valuable and that the fetus is such an organism, or that the fetus is a potential human being and should be protected for that reason (see above for the different views about the human embryo).

- The '*pro-choice*' position: this view holds that ending a pregnancy is a choice that ought to be made by the individual woman involved. The value of the life of the fetus is not seen as zero, but as being subordinate to the rights of the mother to determine what happens to her own body. There are consequentialist and rights-based reasons for this argument:

– consequentialist arguments: some suggested harms that may occur if there was no legal option of a safe termination include:

increasing the poverty of women and their existing children

pregnancy may be a risk to the health of some mothers

women may seek unsafe terminations – putting themselves at even greater risk

– rights-based arguments:

restricting access to abortion is infringement of a woman's autonomy to exercise control over her own body

to refuse an abortion also infringes a woman's right to health and the pursuit of a satisfactory life

(The validity of these arguments in part depends on the acceptance of the 'pro-choice' perspective that fetuses are not human *persons* with rights of their own, or at least not rights that are equivalent in force to those of the pregnant woman.)

The mother–fetus conflict
Clinical dilemma – part I

Miss F has a history of mental disturbance and drug abuse. She is pregnant for a second time – her first child is currently in care. She wishes to continue smoking, drinking and taking drugs throughout this pregnancy. She has not been found to be incompetent. Can the unborn child be made a ward of court in an attempt to curb the mother's harmful behaviour towards it?

This scenario is based on a real case, *Re F (in utero)* [1988] 2 All ER 193; 2 WLR 1288. It is an example of where the autonomy of the mother (to live the lifestyle she wishes) conflicts with the interests of the fetus to be born healthy. Smoking has the potential to cause a number of problems in the baby that will continue outside of the uterus. Excessive alcohol consumption can lead to 'fetal alcohol syndrome', which is characterized by distinctive facies and mental retardation. Drug use may lead to withdrawal symptoms in the fetus and may also be associated with mental retardation.

The courts found that under English law there is no power to curb the woman's behaviour in the interests of the fetus, because until birth the fetus is not a legal person. The *Congenital Disability (Civil Liability) Act* 1976 (as amended by the Human Fertilization and Embryology Act [HFEA] 1990) holds that a mother cannot be held liable for any harm that occurs to the fetus *in utero* (apart from harm due to negligent driving). The courts expressed the view that if the behaviour of pregnant women was to be controlled in order to safeguard the health of their unborn children, this would have to be expressed by an Act of Parliament, rather than the judiciary.

It has been said that if we agree that termination is ethically acceptable, how can we object to harmful behaviour to the fetus that doesn't kill it? However, this objection ignores the difference between a pregnant woman going to term, and a pregnant woman who is going to abort. The former is responsible for harmful consequences to both the fetus *and* the future child. The latter is only responsible for the harmful consequences to the fetus. There is arguably a much greater moral duty upon the woman going to term.

Clearly from a virtue or consequentialist perspective it would be 'better' if Miss F did stop smoking, drinking and taking drugs, not only for the health of her unborn child, but also for her own health. However, this does not necessarily mean that such a moral duty should also be a legal one. Imagine a further development in the scenario.

Clinical dilemma – part II

Miss F is now two weeks past her due date, the baby is in a breech position and is showing signs of fetal distress. It is thought that a caesarean section is the only way of saving the life of the baby. Miss F refuses to have the operation, saying she wants a 'natural' birth. She is still found to be competent. What should her doctor do?

A number of cases have gone to court in order to force women to have caesarean sections – either to preserve their own life, or the life of the unborn child. Legally, if the woman is competent, then her refusal (whatever her reasons) is sufficient to prevent the operation. However, the moral permissibility of refusal may depend on the nature of her reasons. Is it morally permissible for the woman to refuse a caesarean because she doesn't want a scar? What about religious reasons? What about no reason at all?

There is a growing consensus amongst Western clinicians and bioethicists that overriding a competent woman's refusal is almost never justified. The following are a few reasons why:

• Caesareans involve some risk to the mother – the mortality is approximately four times higher than for a vaginal delivery.

- Courts would not order a mother to donate a kidney to an ill child in need of a transplant – so why should they order a caesarean?
- If a woman continued to object, would doctors be expected to forcibly restrain and anaesthetize a pregnant woman?

Sterilization

Ethical and legal issues are most relevant to sterilization when it comes to considering two different things:

1. When can those who cannot consent (for example the mentally incompetent or children) be sterilized?

and

2. Who is responsible if sterilization fails, and a woman becomes pregnant?

Sterilization in the mentally incompetent

As discussed in Chapter 2, consent on behalf of a mentally incompetent adult can only be made if it is in their best interests. With regards to sterilization this leads to an interesting gender bias. Whilst it is arguable that sterilization in mentally incompetent women may be in their best interests, as it prevents the risk of pregnancy, this is not true in men. This gender bias has been reflected in the cases that have gone to court.

The sorts of things that need to be considered, in deciding what is in the patient's best interests include:

- The likelihood of pregnancy – that is, is the individual engaging or likely to engage in sexual intercourse?
- How well is the patient able to understand the concept of pregnancy and its relation to sex?
- Would the patient be able to cope with parenthood?
- Would this patient be able to use any other form of contraception?
- How would a sterilization operation affect the other medical problems of the patient?
- What other support is available to the patient?

Failed sterilization

A number of cases have gone to court when a patient has alleged negligence after a 'failed' sterilization operation that led to a subsequent pregnancy (e.g. *Thake v. Maurice* [1986] 1 All ET 497; *Emeh v. Chelsea & Kensington Area Health Authority* [1984] 3 All ER 1044; *Walkin v. South Manchester Health*

Authority [1995] 4 All ER 132; *Goodwill v. British Pregnancy Advisory Service* [1996] 2 All ER 161). Important points to note are:

- As with other medical negligence cases, information given must be in accordance with a *responsible body of professional practice*.
- In the case of sterilization this means telling the patient both that:
  – the operation is permanent and may be non-reversible

  and

  – there is a failure rate of the operation; that is whilst sterilization is effective, it is not an *absolute guarantee* of never conceiving

Assisted reproduction

The ethical problems surrounding assisted reproduction are numerous. There are problems relating to whether 'infertility' or 'sub-fertility' are 'illnesses', and whether or not they should be treated on the NHS. The answers to this sort of question may turn on whether or not we consider that people have a *right* to have children, and whether such a right applies equally to everyone (including same-sex couples, single women, poor women, women over 40 years or even post-menopausal women).

What then are the different ways in which infertility can be treated?
Gamete donation

This can take the form of egg donation or artificial insemination (AI), either from the husband (AIH) or from a donor (AID). Some of the ethical problems of gamete donation are concerned with:

- The number of children a man can father by AI.
- Whether or not payment can be made for donor sperm or eggs.
- Who is the legal father of the child if donor sperm is used.
- Who is the legal mother of the child when one woman provides the genetic material, and another gives birth to the child.

In vitro fertilization

This requires the fertilization of an egg outside of the human body. It was first successfully carried out in 1978 with the birth of Louise Brown. In-vitro fertilization (IVF) requires the stimulation of ovulation in the woman and the harvesting of eggs. The eggs are incubated with the sperm in a petri dish, and in some cases a single spermatozoon may be injected under the covering of the egg. Finally, the fertilized egg is transferred to the woman's uterus. The ethical problems particular to IVF include:

- The production of excess embryos that must subsequently either be stored (by cryopreservation) or destroyed.
- The increased likelihood of multiple pregnancies and the subsequent increased demand for obstetric and neonatal services.
- The potential for embryo selection to avoid genetic disease, but also potentially to choose the sex, or other characteristics of the embryos.
- Discrimination in the provision of the service against poor, single or older women.

Surrogacy

This can be:

- Partial – in which the surrogate (or carrying) woman's ovum is fertilized by the husband/partner from the commissioning couple, either via IVF, AID or sexual intercourse, so she not only carries the baby, but has a genetic link with it.
- Full – in which the commissioning couple provide both the ovum and the sperm, so that whilst the surrogate carries the child, it is not genetically related to her.

The ethical problems of surrogacy include:

- It represents a separation of genetic, gestational and social parenting.
- It raises the issue of the commodification of human life and the threat of 'baby selling'.
- There are fears of the exploitation and/or coercion of women into being surrogates.

General arguments against in-vitro fertilization and other reproductive technologies are given below.

Assisted reproduction separates sex from reproduction

This argument generally relies on an underlying belief either in natural law theory or a religious principle. A version of natural law theory might claim that the function of sex is reproduction and, therefore, the separation of the two represents an unnatural use of medical technology.

But:

- The problem with this and all '*it's unnatural*' arguments is that nature is not always a good guide in showing what is ethically right and wrong. Much of modern medicine is in a sense unnatural, but this doesn't mean it is *wrong*. Similarly, arguments based on a religious principle are not suitable for basing social policy in a pluralistic society.

Assisted reproduction alters the nature of traditional relationships

IVF and the other reproductive technologies enable single women or lesbian couples to have children. The claim has been made that such individuals are less suitable parents than a heterosexual couple.

But:

- It is yet to be conclusively shown that heterosexual couples are 'better' parents or raise 'better' children, however that may be measured. It is important that children are raised in a loving environment, but it has not been shown that either single parents or same-sex couples are unable to provide such an environment. In the face of such a lack of evidence, we should be cautious in denying the ability to raise children to these sections of society.

Assisted reproduction perpetuates negative social attitudes towards infertile women

This argument runs that there are positive social attitudes towards women who have children, and negative attitudes towards those who either don't have children or don't want children. Such attitudes place pressure on women to become mothers. The presence of IVF and other reproductive technologies increases this pressure. Rather than perpetuate such attitudes the state should encourage acceptance of childlessness within society.

But:

- Whilst there is the possibility of social attitudes factoring in the reasons why a woman might wish for IVF, it is not clear that this would be an overriding reason. Furthermore, it seems to disregard the autonomy of individual women to make the choice for themselves whether or not they would like children.

Assisted reproduction leads to the exploitation of women

IVF is an expensive technology and there have been stories of patients being asked to provide eggs in return for treatment. Furthermore, surrogates have been associated with asking for large sums of money to cover the costs of 'being pregnant'. This argument focuses on the danger of less-well-off women being exploited.

But:

- The plausibility of this argument relies on how one thinks about luxury goods and capitalism in general. Most luxury goods are provided by the less well-off for consumption by the well-off;

whether or not this is exploitation is debatable. What one is obliged to do is to provide full and frank information to all parties about the risks and benefits involved.

Assisted reproduction is not sufficiently important to be provided on the NHS

This argument focuses on the resource issue surrounding the provision of IVF and related services on the NHS. Is it just that people are forced to wait for operations when infertility treatment is being provided? At the time of writing this, the National Institute for Clinical Excellence (NICE) has just issued draft guidance advising that infertile women under 40 should be offered up to six free cycles of IVF. It has been estimated that this will cost £400 million. Is this an appropriate use of resources? Indeed, what obligation, if any, does the NHS have to provide treatment for infertility?

But:

- Being infertile is a profoundly distressing condition for many individuals. Being able to be pregnant, and giving birth and raising a child can be substantial 'goods' in leading a fulfilled life. The provision of IVF *may* lower the associated psychological morbidity of being childless (a matter that could be confirmed empirically – although to the best of my knowledge has not).

Assisted reproduction will lead to eugenic selection

IVF enables embryos to be screened. At present, in the UK this is allowed in order to prevent embryos that will manifest a genetic disease from being implanted. In the case of X-linked diseases, IVF can ensure that only female embryos are implanted. However, the potential exists for sex selection for social reasons. In the future there may be the potential to select embryos on the basis of height, intelligence, sexuality, hair or eye colour. The creation of such 'designer babies' is wrong because it is a eugenic process.

But:

- This argument uses the threat of a *slippery slope* – it implies that by allowing one type of selection now, we will end up with a eugenic programme. However, the fact that we allow some kinds of selection does not mean that we will *inevitably* allow all kinds of selection – this is aptly demonstrated already by the fact that we currently allow sex selection on medical grounds, but not on social grounds.

General ethical approaches to assisted reproduction

A useful way of thinking about the ethics of assisted reproduction is to consider the interests of:

- The (potential) child: for example, what are the consequences to the child of being born to a particular couple? The HFEA 1990 endorses this approach (see below), requiring that account be taken of the '*welfare of any child who may be born*'.
- The parents: is having children who are genetically related a *human right*?
- The state: assisted reproduction is an expensive treatment; are the state's limited resources best spent on this sort of health care? Is infertility a *disease*? Should the state only allow those individuals who are financially capable of supporting a child to have IVF?

Assisted reproduction and legislation

The most important piece of legislation in the area of reproductive medicine is the Human Fertilization and Embryology Act (HFEA) 1990. This was largely based on the 1984 'Report of the Committee of Inquiry into Human Fertilization and Embryology' chaired by the philosopher Mary Warnock (commonly known as the 'Warnock Report').

The HFEA governs:

1. The creation of embryos *in vitro*; i.e. outside the human body.
2. The storage and use of embryos and gametes.

This means it forms the basis for legislation on artificial insemination (in a clinic), egg donation and IVF.

The HFEA 1990 (s. 5) stipulates the creation of the Human Fertilization and Embryology (HF&E) Authority: a body charged with the responsibility of:

1. Keeping under review information about embryos and provision of treatment services and activities governed by the Act.
2. Granting licences to carry out activities specified in the Act to the clinics it deems suitable.
3. Publicising the services provided to the public.
4. Providing appropriate advice to licensed clinics.

Artificial insemination

From the husband (AIH):

- No licence required unless gametes need to be stored or frozen. This usually occurs only if the husband is to undergo treatment that may render him infertile (e.g. chemotherapy).
- Schedule 3 of the HFEA 1990 requires that adequate *written* consent is obtained. It is good

practice for clinics to ensure couples consider what should happen to gametes in relation to:
– the couple splitting up prior to implantation or
– one of the couple dying
– one of the couple losing the capacity to revoke consent
– how long they would like them stored (the 1990 Act stipulated a maximum time limit of ten years for gametes and five years for embryos, although this has now also been extended to ten years).

The case of *R v. HF&E Authority, ex parte Blood* [1996] involved Diane Blood's husband, who had developed meningitis and lapsed into a coma. Diane Blood convinced the doctors treating her husband to remove sperm from her unconscious husband prior to his death: *this act was ILLEGAL* as there was no *written* consent. The sperm were stored at a licensed clinic and thus came within the remit of the HFEA. The HF&E Authority refused her permission to use the sperm in order to conceive a child – even though Diane Blood claimed she and her husband had been trying for a child. The High Court and the Court of Appeal held that insemination in Britain would be illegal. However, the Court of Appeal agreed that under European Law, Diane Blood was entitled to seek medical treatment in another member state. A Belgian clinic agreed to carry out Artificial Insemination, and the HF & E Authority agreed to allow the transport of the sperm to that clinic. However, the Court of Appeal stated that this case should not set a precedent as the taking and storing of the sperm was illegal.

Sperm from a donor (AID):
- Does not always require a licence: all it requires is a suitable male to 'donate' sperm and the woman to self-inseminate; this is often referred to as the 'turkey baster' method or 'do-it-yourself insemination'. If no clinic is involved, it is unregulated. However, *MacLennan v MacLennan* [1958] asks the question of whether such donor insemination constitutes adultery. The courts found that without a sexual relationship it is not.
- Does require a licence when it is done in a clinic under s. 4 of the HFEA 1990.
- Is dealt with in a code of practice issued by HF&E Authority in 1998 covering, amongst other things, the screening of donor gametes. It advised that:
  – screening be carried out for HIV and genetic anomalies (including cystic fibrosis, Tay-Sachs, thalassaemia and sickle cell anaemia)
  – that sperm donors be over 18 years and under 55
  – that egg donors be over 18 years and under 35.
- Must be screened appropriately if used in a clinic setting; s. 44 of the HFEA amends the *Congenital Disabilities Act* making it possible to bring an action against a clinic should negligent screening of gametes take place. Potentially donors can also be liable if they lie about their family/medical history when they donate.
- Is dealt with in ss. 27–29 of the HFEA regarding the parental status of the parties involved:
  – if a married couple have AID, the husband is the legal father
  – if a cohabiting couple both seek AID, the partner is the legal father
  – if a woman receives treatment alone, even if she is in a relationship, there is *no* legal father
  – if treatment occurs outside the remit of the HFEA, for example do-it-yourself inseminations or AID in another country, then the donor becomes the legal father
  – treatment carried out within the remit of the HFEA accords no rights and no responsibilities to the gamete donor.
- Is dealt with under ss. 31–35 of the HFEA regarding the child's right to access information:
  – at 18 an individual who suspects they may have been fathered by donor insemination can find out if their suspicions are true
  – at 16 an individual who wishes to get married and suspects they may have been fathered by donor insemination can find out if they are related to their intended spouse.

In vitro fertilization and gamete intra-fallopian transfer

IVF requires a licence under s. 3 of the HFEA 1990; the conditions relating to storage and use of gametes and embryos are the same as mentioned above. Specifically, ss. 3 and 4 forbid:
- The creation or use of embryos except by licensed clinics.
- Cross-breeding with animals.
- Cloning.
- Use or storage of embryos beyond the formation of the primitive streak; taken to be day 14 of development.
- Germ-cell modification.

Section 13(5) requires clinics to take account of 'the welfare of any child who may be born as a result of the treatment (including the need of that child for a father)'. However, neither the Act nor the Warnock Report on which it was based outlaws the idea of single parents, or lesbian couples, being allowed access to IVF.

Section 38(1) allows for conscientious objection to undergoing the treatment governed by the Act.

GIFT is where the ova and sperm are introduced into the fallopian tubes. Fertilization occurs *in vivo*. Therefore, GIFT is not regulated by the HFEA.

Genetic counselling and screening
Clinical dilemma

A general practitioner cared for a woman during the early stages of Huntington's chorea. Her son, also a patient and aged 48 years, has repeatedly refused any test to establish whether or not he is affected. He remains asymptomatic.

The man is on the point of re-marrying. His fiancée is a 34-year-old woman who also happens to be a patient of the GP, and the GP knows that she desperately wants to have children. The man angrily rejects an invitation from the GP to discuss matters.

The man's daughter from his first marriage is 20 years of age. She too is a patient of the GP. She approaches the GP and asks to be tested for Huntington's chorea before starting a family herself. She does not want her father to know. She does not want the results put in her clinical records as it may affect her application for a life assurance policy.

> Huntington's chorea is a hereditary disease caused by a single gene inherited as a dominant characteristic, tending to appear in 50% of the children of the parents with this condition.
>
> Oxford Concise Colour Medical Dictionary, 1994

We can try to approach this scenario by looking at the duties of care and confidentiality the GP has to each of his patients involved.

The father

The father in the scenario does not wish to be tested. At face value it seems that in order to treat this patient as an autonomous agent, his wishes should be respected. To remain ignorant of his genetic status with regards to Huntington's chorea is a valid stance.
But:

- Respect for autonomy has only prima facie standing. It can be overridden by competing moral obligations, as when respecting someone's autonomy would cause significant harm to

another, i.e. where one person's autonomy inhibits or diminishes that of another. We are told the man is about to re-marry and his fiancée is 'desperate to have children'. So, does the father have any responsibility to tell his fiancée of the increased risk of Huntington's that any of their children may have?

Remember: if the father is a carrier of the Huntington's chorea allele, then any of his children have a 50% chance of inheriting it. He himself has a 50% chance of being a carrier; as his status is unknown, the probability of any of his children being carriers is 1 in 4 or 25%.
However:

- We do not know whether the man wishes to have further children at all. If he doesn't and discusses this with his fiancée and takes the necessary precautions to avoid the situation, there is no reason why the father should be tested or even why he should tell his fiancée of his family history of Huntington's chorea. (Although many would argue he has a duty to his fiancée to be truthful – in order to establish a relationship based on trust.)

- If the man does decide he wishes to have more children with his new wife, and does not inform her of his family history of Huntington's, then the GP is faced with a conflict of moral duties.

The fiancée and future children

The fiancée is one of the GP's patients so the obligation of veracity asks of the GP to be truthful with her. We can assume that the fiancée is keen to be informed of all the possible risks to her children. The GP possesses some information that is relevant to the woman and child, but perhaps ought not to disclose it. Were the woman informed of all the facts she might feel it prudent to have a pre-natal screening done for Huntington's should she fall pregnant. Perhaps by choosing to have further children, in the knowledge that there is a 1 in 4 chance of them being affected by Huntington's, the father's autonomy and thus his right to confidentiality are diminished in favour of the children, as the health and autonomy of third parties are introduced.

The daughter

The daughter is a fully autonomous individual and, therefore, does not require consent from her father to be tested – even though a positive test result will indicate that the father also is positive for

Huntington's. Although he does not wish to know his status, he cannot prevent his daughter from finding out hers. If the daughter is determined to know whether or not she is a carrier of Huntington's, there is no reason why the GP cannot encourage her to discuss the implications of the testing with her father, although if she does not wish to do so, she cannot be coerced into this or have her test made conditional on this.

If her test result is positive for Huntington's, the daughter introduces a greater degree of certainty into the scenario. It will be known to both the daughter and the GP that the man is also a carrier and thus any future child of the man will have a 50% chance of developing Huntington's. The daughter now possesses knowledge about her own condition that implies information about her father's genetic status. Her father has no rights over this knowledge – it is information that is 'owned' by his daughter. The father's right to privacy has been curtailed because of the third parties involved and the fact that his carrier status is deduced via a test on relatives rather than actually on him. For the daughter to discuss this with her father's fiancée could be seen as a breach of his privacy, although perhaps the fiancée's right to be informed overrides this. This right to be informed, however, may not override the GP's duty of confidentiality, so it may be that there is less of a moral dilemma if the daughter informs the fiancée of her family history of Huntington's rather than the GP doing it. With regards to situations like this, John Harris says that 'While it will always be open to individuals to refuse tests for themselves, they may not be able to so effectively shield themselves from the increased knowledge of their own chances, which will come from relatives who do opt for the test. They will also have to consider whether they are justified in having children who will certainly, or probably, have the disease' (Harris 1994). This shows that the greatest responsibility lies with the father – it is he who must decide if he is justified in having children that may have Huntington's.

The end of the scenario mentions the daughter's wish for the test not to be recorded on her clinical records as it might adversely affect her life insurance. If the test is done, it seems important that it is recorded. There is no reason for the GP to break any confidences and inform any insurer – it is up to the patient what information they give to the insurer. On a broader scale we can ask whether genetic screening should cause people to be liable for higher insurance premiums. If we are happy for this to occur with

other diseases such as familial heart disease and diabetes, should genetic tests not be just as acceptable? This debate would of course depend on the reliability of such tests.

Gene therapy and cloning (adapted from Amarakone & Capps)

On February 23, 1997, aged just six months, Dolly the sheep was revealed to the world's media by the Roslin Institute, Edinburgh. Dolly had been cloned directly from a single cell from the breast tissue of an adult sheep. Six years later, Dolly had to be put down as she was suffering from a type of lung disease that normally affects sheep at around the age of 11 or 12 years. The suggestion was made that this 'premature ageing' was a result of the cloning process. This news has cast a shadow over those who claim that human cloning is both feasible and desirable.

That same year, the UNESCO *Declaration on the Human Genome and Human Rights*, as signed by 186 nations, stated 'practices such as the reproductive cloning of human beings shall not be permitted'. In December 2001 the UK Parliament passed the *Human Reproductive Cloning Act* to make human cloning illegal. Given this apparent consensus against cloning, how as medics should we approach the ethical debate?

One starting point is a variation of Mill's Liberty Principle. We can reasonably extend the principle that individuals should be free to act as they please, as long as their actions don't harm anyone, to the act of reproduction. Along these lines, John Harris talks of a 'procreative autonomy'. This is the idea that individuals should be allowed to control and exercise choice with regard to how they reproduce. Such a freedom is especially important when the choices made cause little harm to either the children produced or society as a whole, and in addition extends a principle such as respect for autonomy. In essence, this argument, when applied to the question of cloning, requires that in order to restrict choice and freedom we present a strong case as to why cloning is unacceptable.

One way of doing this may be to claim that cloning in fact causes *significant* harm to children, that cloning is fundamentally an 'unsafe' technology. Dolly died aged six, even though the expected lifespan of a sheep is about 12 years. There is a chance that human clones would have a similarly foreshortened life. In addition to the risk of premature death in successful cloning attempts, there is the problem of producing large numbers of malformed embryos. Reproductive cloning could lead to the birth of an unacceptably high number of disabled infants, many of which would not be able to survive without significant pain and suffering, or necessitate a large number of terminations. The potential to recklessly produce individuals that suffer may well be sufficient grounds to ban all reproductive human cloning. However, if cloning could be carried out without such risks, would any objections still exist? That is, what, if anything, is *intrinsically* wrong with cloning humans? The following are a few commonly given suggestions.

Cloning is wrong because:
- It prevents genetic variation.
- It is unnatural.
- It deprives clones of the right to be unique.
- It would be a psychological harm to those born as a result of it.
- It treats children as commodities.

The loss of genetic variation argument

The loss of genetic variation argument runs that sexual reproduction is essential in producing variation within the human species; cloning removes this variation and, thus, reduces genetic diversity – this may in the long-term threaten the survival of the species.

But:
- It is likely that only a tiny minority of people would ever use cloning technology, and this surely would not be sufficient to threaten species survival.
- Even if everyone in the world were to be cloned, genetic diversity would not change from what it is now – in fact it would stay exactly the same. (This assumes that only one clone of each person is made.)

However, problems involving reduced diversity could arise if some individuals produce vast numbers of clones, for example if a 'crazy dictator' decides to create clone armies.

But:
- This objection is really to do with a misuse of a technology rather than an objection to the technology itself. Baseball bats can be used when mugging someone, but this doesn't mean we should ban baseball.

If cloning were to be used, then it would have to be regulated, as IVF and abortion are currently regulated. At the root of this sort of concern may be the fear that once we allow certain procedures that involve tampering with the human genome, there is a slippery slope to full-blown eugenic policies being introduced. This type of concern affects a number of genetic techniques, including sex selection, pre-natal genetic diagnosis and selective terminations.

The 'it's unnatural' argument

A more common accusation is that cloning is 'unnatural' – it arouses a feeling of uneasiness that cannot easily be clarified. This is sometimes called the 'yuck factor'. It is perhaps encapsulated by the idea that cloning involves 'playing God'. Indeed, some religious commentators have opposed cloning on the grounds that clones would be born without souls because they are lives created by man rather than by God. While it may be difficult to see why this is the case, the definitive rebuttal of such religious arguments is problematic simply because questions of faith exist beyond logical argument. It is, however, easier to tackle the thought that cloning is 'unnatural'. It seems that much of modern medicine is, in a sense, 'unnatural'. Heart transplants are a prime example of an 'unnatural' procedure. They involve the removal of the heart from a brain-dead body that is being kept alive artificially and its insertion into the body of another individual. However, 'unnatural' does not always mean 'morally wrong'. An objection to cloning must involve something over and above a sense of being unnatural, or simply prompting a sense of disgust. The crux of the 'it's unnatural' argument may be to defend the notion that technological developments should be used in such a way as to improve humanity without destroying or detracting from what it is to be 'human'.

Clones are not 'unique'

What then of the 'right' to be unique? Can clones be unique if they are 'copies' of other people? We know that identical twins have identical copies of DNA, and at the same time they exist as unique individuals with differing personalities. If we think of clones as 'vertical twins', rather than 'horizontal' ones, there is no reason to suppose that they will be any less unique from their vertical twins than identical twins are from their horizontal twins. In fact, given the different environments in which they are raised we could suppose that clones would be rather more different than horizontal twins are.

Psychological harm to the clone

Next, there are those who object to human cloning on the grounds of the harm that might be inflicted on the child. Indeed, the HFEA, which governs IVF treatment and the use of embryos, indicates that the *good of the child is paramount*. The sentiment of the Act is clear, but what exactly is the nature of the harm that may be visited upon a clone? The harm is often described as psychological and may have at least two aspects.

First, there is said to be the burden a child would have of seeing exactly how they would appear at various ages, by seeing photographs (or home videos) of their 'parent' at those ages. The problem with this objection is that there simply isn't any evidence for it. Many sons already look at their balding fathers and resign themselves to the same fate, without suffering too greatly for it. Similarly, daughters may see their mother's nose or eyes in their own countenance and either cherish or bemoan that fact, without suffering undue harm. Granted, the similarity will be greater between clones, but the idea that that fact will lead to *intolerable* suffering, such that we consider it is better that child doesn't exist, is unsubstantiated.

Second, there is the objection that the 'parents' may expect too much of their clones. For example, a concert pianist may clone himself and expect (to an unreasonable degree) his clone to possess a similar talent for music. However, many parents may place unreasonable demands on their children in this way. The children of doctors often feel pressurized into medical careers, but no-one suggests that doctors don't have children; what they suggest is that children be accorded the freedom to flourish in areas of their own choosing. There is no reason to suspect that the 'parents' of clones will be unable to accord their 'children' such a freedom. They may be more likely to expect too much of them (because of certain preconceptions), but this is not an *inevitable* consequence of cloning. Thus any harm that is isolated, if it exists, is located in the parenting not the act of cloning. Indeed, it may be that a *planned* child which is cloned may be more cherished than one conceived accidentally.

The commodification of children

Finally, there is the objection that cloning represents a commodification of children and this in itself is wrong. Implicit in this claim is that there is no morally admirable reason for producing a clone. The standard reason given for wanting to clone oneself is that cloning represents the only chance that a particular individual can have a genetically related child. The strength of this reason depends on whether we consider that people can be said to have a *right* to have genetically related children. The fact

that, from an evolutionary perspective, the purpose of living can be said to be reproduction is ethically neither here nor there. Nature is not a good guide in matters of morality. Thus, is the desire to have a genetically related child simply a selfish one – a desire that treats children simply as a consumer product? Is there in any sense a health-care *need* for cloning that cannot be satisfied by the reproductive technologies already available? Tied in with this question is that of what kind of person would desire to have a clone? And, are they the kind of people who should be able to have clones? It may be that whilst cloning *in principle* is morally acceptable (that is for *good* purposes), *in practice* the only people who would want clones would want them for morally unacceptable reasons (for example *unreasonably* wanting to replace a dead child).

Children

The rights of children

In 1989 the UN introduced the International Convention on the Rights of the Child. This endowed children with the rights to self-determination, dignity and respect. The European Charter for Children in Hospital states 'Children and parents have the right to informed participation in all decisions involving their health care. Every child shall be protected from unnecessary medical treatment and investigation' (McHale et al. 1997). The idea of the 'rights of children' has certainly been increasing over the past 15 years; however, it is not universally accepted. The concept of being paternalistic is obviously stronger in the treatment of children because children are thought to be less autonomous than adults. That is, their ability to understand their health status and use that information to give a considered decision, in accordance with their life goals, is assumed to be inferior to that of an adult. Such an ability is thought to develop only as a young child grows and matures. The purpose of the 'rights of children' has been to prevent excessive paternalism: to ensure that physicians and parents recognize the developing autonomy of children. Some philosophers have thought it unhelpful to talk of children's rights – rather that it is more prudent to talk about the obligations of parents. However, as Western culture becomes more focused on individual rights (rather than duties), it seems that the notion of the 'rights of children' is here to stay.

The Children Act 1989

This act is relevant in a number of ways:

1. It asserts that the welfare of the child is of *paramount importance* in court decisions about the future of the child.
2. It outlines who has parental responsibility for a child and how to make decisions where those with parental responsibility disagree.
3. It outlines the arrangements that can be made in order to protect a child from harm or to provide care in the event of those with parental responsibility being unable to.

The Act provides a checklist (s. 1(3)) in order to guide the decisions made by the courts:

- A court should have regard in particular to:
  - the wishes and feelings of the child concerned (dependent on age and understanding)
  - the physical, emotional and educational needs of the child
  - the likely effect of any change on the child
  - the age, sex, background and any other relevant characteristic of the child
  - any harm this child has suffered or is at risk of suffering
  - the capability of each parent in meeting the needs of the child
  - the range of powers available to the court.

Children and consent

In law a child is any individual under 18 years old. This is defined by the *Children Act 1989* (s. 105). Those with parental responsibility can consent to medical treatment on behalf of a child – regardless of the child's consent. However, it would be rare to treat a competent 17-year-old who refused treatment solely on the grounds of the parental consent (Fig. 3.2).

Fraser competence

The authoritative case in relation to children and consent was the *Gillick* case. Mrs Gillick had 10 children, a number of whom were girls under the age of 16. She was concerned by a Department of Health and Social Security circular that advocated the preservation of confidentiality when the patient was requesting contraception, even if the patient was less than 16 years old.

Mrs Gillick objected and went to court to ensure that the Health Authority did not give contraceptive advice to her children without her consent. The case went all the way to the House of Lords, which decided against Mrs Gillick. It was asserted that:

- The parental right to 'control a child' existed for the benefit of the child not the parent; it was thus only justified in the best interests of the child.
- The parental right should yield to the child's right when the child reaches a sufficient understanding and intelligence.
- The sufficient understanding and intelligence may be present in a child under the age of 16 years; it is up to the doctor to assess whether the child is capable of understanding the medical, social and moral aspects of the proposed treatment.

Lord Fraser produced a check-list approach, which included that:

- The girl understood the advice given, including the possible consequences.
- The doctor was unable to convince the girl to inform her parents.
- The girl would have intercourse with or without contraception (this avoided the charge of aiding and abetting sex with a minor).
- Without contraception there was a likelihood of mental or physical harm.
- It was in the best interests of the child not to have parental consent.

This judgement allows only mature children under the age of 16 to *consent* to medical treatment, it does not allow them to *refuse*. In fact, *refusal* is not binding until the age of 18 (Figs 3.3, 3.4).

The term 'Gillick Competence' was in wide use until a recent complaint from Mrs Gillick led to it being dropped in favour of the current usage, which refers instead to Lord Fraser.

Child abuse

Child abuse includes:

- Physical abuse.
- Emotional abuse.
- Sexual abuse.
- Neglect.

Medical professionals may become involved with cases of child abuse as a result of:

- A member of the public reporting their suspicions about abuse.
- Treating a child.
- Being asked by the local authority to investigate a child for evidence of abuse.

If abuse is suspected, a *senior doctor should be consulted*, preferably one with expertise in child abuse, before making allegations or reporting the suspicions to other agencies. This is because an

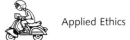

Children and consent

Age group	Who can consent to treatment		Who can refuse treatment	
Under 16 years	*Patient*	Yes – if Fraser competent	*Patient*	No
	Parents	Yes	*Parents*	Yes – but doctors can appeal to courts, who can overturn refusal
	Courts	Yes	*Courts*	Yes – although unlikely to disagree with medical opinion
	Doctors	Yes – if no-one with parental responsibility is available, doctors can treat in the best interests of the child	*Doctors*	Yes – doctors retain the right not to treat patients if they believe this is in the best interests of the patient or they have a conscientious objection (in which case they should refer to another doctor). Doctors must treat in emergencies (if in the patient's best interests)
16–18-year-olds	*Patient*	Yes – presumed competent to consent	*Patient*	No – refusal can be overridden by parents or by the courts
	Parents	Yes – even if the child refuses	*Parents*	Yes – but overridden if child or the courts consent
	Courts	Yes	*Courts*	Yes
	Doctors	Yes – if no-one with parental responsibility is available, in an emergency, doctors can treat in the best interests	*Doctors*	Yes – doctors retain the right not to treat patients if they believe this is in the best interests of the patient or they have a conscientious objection (in which case they should refer to another doctor). Doctors must treat in emergencies (if in the patient's best interests)
>18 years	*Patient*	Yes	*Patient*	Yes
	Parents	No	*Parents*	No
	Courts	No – unless patient is incompetent, then courts can decide what is in the patient's best interests	*Courts*	Yes
	Doctors	No – unless patient is incompetent, then doctors can treat in the patient's best interests. If the doctors are unclear as to what a patient's best interests are, they can refer the decision to the courts	*Doctors*	Yes – doctors retain the right not to treat patients if they believe this is in the best interests of the patient or they have a conscientious objection (in which case they should refer to another doctor). Doctors must treat in emergencies (if in the patient's best interests)

Fig. 3.2 Children and consent.

incorrect allegation of abuse can be devastating for families and inappropriate examinations can be devastating for the child.

The responsibility for investigating abuse lies primarily with the local authority. However, a number of agencies are involved. These include social services, doctors, nurses, and the police. If the local authority requests the help of a doctor, the doctor is obliged to co-operate. As mentioned before, the welfare of the child is of paramount importance.

Consent and developing competence

Explanation: appropriate for use with children of *any* age – talking in a soothing manner may help to reassure any child, regardless of their verbal ability

Assent: should be sought from any child that can understand the purpose of treatment:
6–7-year-olds may view treatment as punishment
7–10-year-olds may begin to understand the need for treatment, but not necessarily why it may be painful
10–12-year-olds may start to take a more mature approach to treatment – understanding that investigations may be painful, but beneficial in the long run
12–14-year-olds may be able to satisfy *Fraser* competence

Consent:
14–16-year-olds is the age group to which *Fraser* competence is most likely to apply
16+ capacity to consent is presumed

Note: Where there is fluctuating capacity in a child, the child is assessed with respect to their capacity when they are at the *least lucid*, i.e. on *bad* days. This is inconsistent with the approach to adults where it is the capacity at the time of the act that is relevant

---

Fig. 3.3 Consent and developing competence.

Who has parental responsibility?

Knowing who has parental responsibility is important for health-care professionals as it is only these individuals who can consent to medical assessment and treatment if the child is unable to do so. Although a number of people may have parental responsibility, a doctor requires consent from only one individual. The following individuals have parental responsibility:

• The mother

• The father – if currently married to the mother or was married to the mother at the time of insemination or at birth

• If not married to the mother, the father can acquire parental responsibility by:
 – a written agreement with the mother
 – a court order
 – being appointed the child's guardian after the mother's death

• Adoptive parents – in this case the original parents cease to have parental responsibility

• Guardians – parents may appoint a person(s) to be responsible for their children after their death

• A person obtaining a residence order (by which a child is placed in their care – often with grandparents or other relatives) will also usually obtain parental responsibility. The original parents do not lose parental responsibility

• A local authority named in a care order – again the original parents do not lose parental responsibility

---

Source: adapted with permission from Hope T, Salvulescu J, Hendrick J 2003 Medical Ethics and Law. Edinburgh, Churchill Livingstone, pp. 135–136

Fig. 3.4 Who has parental responsibility?

Child protection orders

The Children Act 1989 gives power to the courts to issue a number of different orders that aim to safeguard children.

Specific issue order

This addresses a specific question that is in dispute. The courts will resolve the issue by saying what they think should be done. For example, if parents and doctors disagree about the treatment a child should receive, the courts will consider the question and decide one way or the other (usually in favour of the doctors).

Care and supervision order

The courts may make this order to place a child at risk of harm, or suffering actual harm, in the care of a local authority and to give parental authority to the local authority.

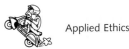

Emergency protection order

This is issued where there is an urgent need to move a child at risk to a safe place.

Child assessment order

This allows a court to have a child, believed to be at risk, assessed by a doctor for evidence of abuse. However, if the child is of sufficient understanding, the child can refuse to submit to any such medical or psychiatric assessment.

Mental disorder and disability

Psychiatric ethics is in a different class from ethics in other fields of medicine. Some of the reasons for this are:
- Psychiatrists wield a great deal of power over patients through the ability to section – that is detain patients in hospital – against their will.
- Unlike the rest of medicine, patients may commonly be incompetent; thus, the bedrock of Western ethics, patient autonomy, appears less stable a foundation from which to base ethical reasoning.
- Psychological therapy enhances the general power divide between doctor and patient, by encouraging patients to reveal highly personal and intimate details about their life.
- Powerful psychopharmacological treatment can be used to change the personality, and perhaps the identity of patients.
- Historically, the mentally ill have been a vulnerable section of society. Even today media portrayal of the mentally ill is predominantly negative leading to stigma and increased isolation of the mentally ill community.
- A lack of clarity over the nature of mental illness. Psychiatrists such as Thomas Szasz and RD Laing have to different degrees criticized the notion that mental illness has a physical or biological basis – sometimes describing many of the disorders as 'problems of living' rather than disease.

Psychiatric codes of ethics

The first ethical code specific to psychiatry was drawn up in 1973 by the American Psychiatric Association. Following this the World Psychiatric Association launched a code in 1977 at its World Congress in Honolulu known as the *Declaration of Hawaii*. This was updated as the *Declaration of Madrid* in 1996. These are some of the principles :

1. Psychiatrists should devise therapeutic interventions that are the least restrictive to the freedom of the patient.
2. The patient should be accepted as partner in the therapeutic process.
3. It is the duty of psychiatrists to provide the patient with relevant information to enable the patient to come to a rational decision according to his or her personal values and preferences.
4. When the patient is incapacitated and /or unable to exercise proper judgement because of a mental disorder, the psychiatrist should consult with the family, and, if appropriate, seek legal counsel in order to safeguard the patient's dignity and legal rights.
5. No treatment should be imposed against the patient's will *unless* doing so endangers the life of the patient *and/or* those who surround him.
6. Treatment must always be in the best interest of the patient.
7. Breach of confidentiality may only be appropriate to prevent serious mental or physical harm to the patient *or* a third party.

The Mental Health Act 1983

The Mental Health Act (MHA) 1983 is the most important piece of legislation dealing with the treatment of mentally ill individuals. (It is, however, currently under review.) The MHA represents an exception to the generally accepted rule that adults must consent to treatment. The MHA primarily deals with compulsory detention of patients in psychiatric hospitals; however, it does also cover the enforcement of treatment outside hospitals.

There are two main ethical justifications for the compulsory detention of people:
1. To protect patients from harming themselves.
2. To protect patients from harming others.

Compulsory admission is governed by two sections of the MHA:
- **Section 2** allows for admission for the purpose of *assessment* – it cannot exceed 28 days. Patients can be admitted if:
  – the patient is 'suffering from mental disorder of a nature or degree that warrants the detention of the patient'.

and
  – the patient ought to be so detained in the interests of his own health or safety or with a view to the protection of other persons.

– admission is supported by two registered medical practitioners (often the psychiatrist and the patient's GP) and an approved social worker or relative.

- **Section 3** allows for admission for the purpose of *treatment* – which in the first instance should not be for longer than six months (this can be extended after review first for another six months, then for one year at a time). Patients can be admitted if:
  - the patient is suffering from mental illness, severe mental impairment, psychopathic disorder or mental impairment of 'a nature or degree which makes it appropriate for him to receive medical treatment in a hospital'
  - in the case of psychopathic disorder or mental impairment, 'such treatment is likely to alleviate or prevent a deterioration of his condition'; this is known as the 'treatability requirement'; patients cannot be detained simply to protect themselves or others, rather there must be some treatment available. This criterion in particular has come under review in the Draft Mental Health Bill released in June 2002. The draft bill proposes to allow the indefinite detention of those patients who are diagnosed with personality disorders and who are a risk to others.
  - it is for the protection of the health and safety of the patient or for the protection of others

  - treatment cannot be provided unless the patient is detained
  - admission is supported by two registered medical practitioners (often the psychiatrist and the patient's GP) and an approved social worker or relative.

In addition special note is made that patients cannot be detained on the grounds of:
- Dependence on drugs and/or alcohol.
- Promiscuity.
- Sexual deviancy (Fig. 3.5).

The Draft Mental Incapacity Bill 2003, which may be called the Mental Capacity Act when it is passed, had the following key points:
- This Act *only* concerns those who are legally incapable.
- Capacity is not present if a person is:
  - unable to understand relevant information.

  or
  - unable to retain the relevant information.

  or
  - unable to use the information to come to a decision.

  or
  - unable to communicate the decision.

The Mental Health Act 1983

The Mental Health Act is *only* applicable to those with a *mental disorder* and can only be used to treat that mental disorder – not to treat other physical disorders that the patient may have

Clearly the key term used is *mental disorder* – but what exactly constitutes a mental disorder? The MHA states that mental disorder includes:

1. *Mental illness* – it does not further define this; however, the meaning of this term has been considered by the courts where it was stated ' . . . there is no definition of "mental illness". The words are ordinary words of the English language . . . [and] should be construed in the way that ordinary sensible people would construe them' (W v. L [1974] QB 711, [1973] 3 WLR 859). This has been called 'the man must be mad' test (Hoggett 1996). A DHSS consultation document stated that mental illness was characterized by: more than temporary impairment of intellectual functions; delusions; abnormal perceptions; and disordered thinking (i.e. effectively psychosis)

2. *Severe mental impairment* – 'a state of arrested or incomplete development of mind which includes severe impairment of intelligence and social functioning and is associated with abnormally aggressive or seriously irresponsible conduct on the part of the person concerned' – that is learning disabilities with aggressive or irresponsible conduct
   Note: learning disabilities by themselves are not sufficient grounds to detain individuals against their will

3. *Mental impairment* – 'a state of arrested or incomplete development of mind (not amounting to severe mental impairment) which includes significant impairment of intelligence and social functioning and is associated with abnormally aggressive or seriously irresponsible conduct on the part of the person concerned'

4. *Psychopathic disorder* – 'a persistent disorder or disability of mind (whether or not including significant impairment of intelligence) which results in abnormally aggressive or seriously irresponsible conduct on the part of the person concerned'

5. *Any other disorder or disability of mind* – this is not defined by the Act

Fig. 3.5 The Mental Health Act 1983.

- All decisions made on behalf of a person who lacks capacity must be done in their best interests (see Consent p. 18 for what constitutes 'best interests').
- It introduces the concept of 'general authority', which allows a carer to make decisions about money, health and care for someone who is unable to make those decisions themselves. (The scope of general authority is restricted by 'best interests'.)
- It encourages the use of independent advocates to speak on behalf of the incapacitated person.
- It allows people to choose a person to whom they give 'lasting power of attorney' or LPA. LPA allows decisions to be made about health, wealth and social care; however, the person who is choosing the LPA decides what decisions the LPA can make. Usually this will be done in advance of a person becoming incapacitated, for example a patient in the early stages of Alzheimer's may decide who should be able to make decisions on their behalf when they are no longer capable and on what they may make those decisions. However, a person with LPA must still consider the incapacitated person's best interests.
- The Bill will create a new 'Court of Protection' that will make decisions on behalf of those without capacity. Decisions on financial and social care as well as medical care will be made. (Decisions on medical care are currently made in the High Court.)
- The Court of Protection will have the power to make a court-appointed deputy to make decisions on the incapacitated person's behalf: this will usually be a relative or friend.
- 'Public Guardians' will be charged with the responsibility of ensuring that court-appointed deputies are acting within the law.
- The Bill proposes to legitimize advance directives or advance decisions:
  - an 'advance decision' means a decision made by a person over the age of 18, whilst that person has capacity, which consents to or refuses a specified treatment that may or may not be carried out, at a time when that person is no longer capable of making such treatment decisions
  - advance decisions must be 'valid' and 'applicable':
    advance decisions are invalid if the person has withdrawn the decision at a time whilst capable of doing so, has given a LPA permission to make decisions about the advance decision, or done anything inconsistent with the advance decision being a fixed decision
    advance decisions are not applicable if the treatment proposed is not the one specified by the advance decision, or if any circumstances specified in the advance decision are absent, or if circumstances that the person did not envisage and that may have affected that person's decision are present
    advance decisions are not applicable to a life-sustaining treatment unless explicitly specified in the advance directive.

The ethics of involuntary treatment

Competence refers to the patient's ability to understand, deliberate, make rational choices and communicate them to the doctor. The legal standard for competence (which is synonymous with capacity) was set out by the *Re C* test (see Chapter 2).

When a patient is judged to be incompetent, they are treated according to what is thought to be in their *best interests*. As mentioned above, the ethical justification for involuntary treatment is to prevent harm to either the patient or others. Arguments for and against involuntary treatment are summarized below (adapted from Peele & Chodoff 1999).

Those who maintain mental illness is a myth argue that people with such 'problems' – whilst they should receive treatment if they so wish – should not be forced to have treatment as they do not recognize mental illness as a 'real' disease. The most prominent advocate of this argument was Thomas Szasz. Szasz considered mental disorders to be 'problems with living' – dependent on the environment or individual reaction to stressors – without a biological cause.

But:

- It has become progressively more difficult to maintain the assertion that mental illness is a myth given what is now known about the biological correlates of illnesses such as depression and schizophrenia and their responsiveness to psychotropic drugs.

Others who accept mental illness as a real phenomenon argue that psychiatric treatment is only effective when the patient consents to treatment. This view holds that coercion is never justified in the treatment of the mentally ill.

But:

- This ignores the effectiveness of coercion in some situations. An analogy could be drawn with an ill child who refuses treatment because he fears needles. Mental illness can reduce some individuals to a similar child-like state, where long-term goals are not considered. In addition, experience shows that many patients who are coerced into treatment are grateful for such treatment after recovery, even if they refused treatment at the time.

A final group believe that the reasons for patients not consenting to treatment should be addressed prior to enforcing involuntary treatment. This would include reducing the social stigma of being institutionalized in a psychiatric hospital, and making such places more accessible and more inviting to stay.
But:

- It seems unlikely that the stigma of mental illness can be entirely eradicated (although this doesn't mean we shouldn't try).

Patient, family and community

One area in which the rights of mentally ill patients conflict with those of the public at large is that of confidentiality. What should a psychiatrist do if a mentally ill patient reveals to them (under the assumption of confidentiality) a desire to harm other people? Such a situation was addressed in the following case.

Case discussion

Tarasoff v. Regents of the University of California, 17 Cal. 3d 425. The facts:

- A patient attending the University of California student health centre revealed to a psychologist that he intended to harm another student, Ms Tarasoff, who had rejected his advances.
- The psychologist did not detain the patient even though the patient was considered to be a serious risk to others.
- Ms Tarasoff was not informed of the potential danger to herself.
- The patient attacked and killed Ms Tarasoff.
- The parents of Ms Tarasoff successfully sued the psychologist for not breaking confidentiality and informing Ms Tarasoff.

The judgements in favour of maintaining confidentiality include the following:

1. Deterrence from treatment – without the assurance of confidentiality 'those requiring treatment will be deterred from seeking assistance'.
2. Full disclosure – the 'guarantee of confidentiality is essential in eliciting the full disclosure necessary for effective treatment'.
3. Successful treatment – confidentiality is an integral part of procuring a successful treatment; trust between patient and physician or therapist is essential.
4. Violence and civil commitment – without confidentiality treatment will suffer as outlined above, and thus the violence committed by those who are mentally ill will increase. Furthermore, the risk of civil commitment of the mentally ill, 'the total deprivation of liberty', will increase. Justice Clark (who outlined the minority opinion *Tarasoff v. Regents of the University of California*) claimed that 'although under existing psychiatric procedures only a relatively few receiving treatment will ever present a risk of violence, the number making threats is huge, and it is the latter group – not just the former – whose treatment will be impaired and whose risk of commitment will be increased'.

The judgements in favour of disclosure include the following:

1. The therapist–patient relationship – in general, under common law, no-one is responsible for the conduct of another nor under a duty to warn those endangered by such conduct. But, where a 'special relationship' exists between an individual and the person whose conduct needs to be controlled, or the foreseeable victim of that conduct, there is an exception to this general rule. The therapist–patient relationship was found to satisfy this relationship.
2. Autonomy of the victim – given that the duty of confidentiality is based on a respect for autonomy, we should also consider the loss of autonomy of the victim and weigh that against the loss of autonomy (to the patient) caused by disclosure, even if unwarranted. Justice Tobriner did this in the Tarasoff case and stated: 'the risk that unnecessary warnings may be given is a reasonable price to pay for the lives of possible victims that may be saved'.
3. Public interest in disclosure – the Tarasoff case asserted that there existed a public interest in the maintenance of confidences, but that this could be outweighed by a public interest in safety from attack.

The end of life

The treatment of those with terminal illnesses is perhaps one of the most distressing fields of medicine. The ethical questions in this area not only include when it is appropriate to stop treatment, but also what forms (if any) of euthanasia are justifiable and how to approach the question of organ donation. The ethical questions are not so much of a different kind, but they are different in degree, because often it is life itself that is at stake.

Euthanasia

The Greek roots of the word 'euthanasia' mean a 'good death' and are thus suggestive that 'euthanasia' is a welcome practice. However, this may not be so simple to decide. Euthanasia is now almost entirely understood to be an action or omission by a doctor that leads to the death of a patient. There are understood to be a number of different types of euthanasia:

- Voluntary euthanasia: euthanasia is *requested* by a patient who is *fully informed* and *competent* and is carried out for the patient's benefit.
- Non-voluntary euthanasia: euthanasia is carried out on a patient who is *not* competent (for example a PVS patient).
- Involuntary euthanasia: euthanasia on a competent patient who does not wish to die.

Euthanasia can be either:

- Active – this involves *killing the patient* by doing some *action* that leads to the death of the patient, for example giving the patient a lethal injection. Active euthanasia is illegal and would be classified as murder.
- Passive – this is *allowing a patient to die*; it may involve:
  - withholding treatment – for example a 'do not attempt resuscitation' order (DNAR)
  - withdrawing treatment – for example stopping a ventilator.

Passive euthanasia is not necessarily illegal, as long as it is in the best interests of the patient. So where there is evidence, or medical consensus, that aggressive resuscitation is ineffective in certain patients then a DNAR may be appropriate. Similarly the removal of medical care may be permissible if it is not in the patient's best interests to continue receiving such care.

Do not attempt resuscitation orders

The do not attempt resuscitation order (DNAR) involves making an advance decision to withhold care from a patient, in the event that they require cardio-respiratory resuscitation. Resuscitation is like any other treatment, so a DNAR should be considered only when:

- Resuscitation is *not* in the best interests of the patient; that is, it is likely to cause a quality of life that is considered to be worse than death.
- Resuscitation is likely to be *futile*.
- Resuscitation is contrary to the informed wishes of a competent patient; that is, resuscitation is not *consented to*.
- Resuscitation is contrary to an *advance directive*.

The law and euthanasia

The law in general supports the idea of autonomy; however, the courts have never claimed that this leads to a 'right to die' that is sufficiently powerful to allow doctors to participate in active euthanasia. It remains indisputably *illegal* to actively administer a fatal injection with the intention of killing a patient, regardless of whether the patient has consented to such an injection and regardless of whether such an injection would constitute a 'mercy killing'. However, the courts have shown a tendency to be lenient with such cases. In contrast the courts have been willing to sanction cases of non-treatment or withdrawal of care leading to death, both in neonates and in adults.

Important cases in the development of case law on euthanasia
Active euthanasia

In the case of *R v. Arthur* [1981], Dr Arthur, a paediatrician, prescribed DF118 to a newly born infant with Down's syndrome and no other complications. He wrote in the notes 'Parents do not wish child to survive. For nursing care only.' The effect of this was to set the conditions in which the child developed pneumonia and then died. Dr Arthur was originally charged with murder, then attempted murder, but was acquitted of all charges. It was held that non-treatment was not murder because it was an *omission* rather than an *act*. However, this is widely accepted as a misapplication of the law as an omission can be grounds for murder if there is *duty of care*, which there clearly was. It is unlikely that a similar case today would result in an acquittal.

In the case of *R v. Carr* [1986], Dr Carr was charged with murder of a terminally ill adult after he administered a massive dose of phenobarbitone. Although Dr Carr was acquitted, the judgement held that 'every patient was entitled to every hour that God had given him, however seriously ill he might be'.

In the case of *R v. Cox* [1992], Dr Cox gave a 70-year-old woman with rheumatoid arthritis and multiple other pathologies an injection of potassium chloride (on her request). He was charged with murder and given a one-year suspended prison sentence. The GMC warned him, but allowed him to continue practice, as it believed him to have acted in good faith.

Painkillers and the doctrine of double effect In the case of *R v. Bodkin Adams* [1957], Dr Adams was tried for murder after the death of a patient who had made him a beneficiary of her will. He had prescribed heroin and morphine to an 80-year-old woman following a stroke. It was not the first patient who had left him items in their wills. The judge in this case held that:

> The defence in the present case was that the treatment given by Dr Adams was designed to promote comfort, and if it was the right and proper treatment, the fact that it shortened life did not convict him of murder.

This is held to be the first court approval of the doctrine of double effect (see below for a discussion of the moral aspects of this doctrine).

Passive euthanasia
Neonates There have been a number of cases where disabled newborns have had treatment withdrawn or withheld. The courts have tended to take the approach that aggressive treatment for gravely handicapped children need not be pursued, especially if there is only a short gain in life expectancy anticipated from treatment.

Adults In the case of *Airedale NHS Trust v. Bland* [1993] Tony Bland was injured at the Hillsborough football ground in April 1989 after being crushed in the crowd. He was diagnosed as being in a persistent vegetative state (PVS) with no signs of recovery. He was not ventilated, but was fed via a naso-gastric tube. The hospital treating him sought court approval to discontinue treatment. His family agreed that treatment should be withdrawn. This case went all the way to the House of Lords.

Lord Goff gave the leading judgement. He started from the premise that Tony Bland was still alive. He considered the 'sanctity of life' arguments, but decided they were not absolute, and that 'sanctity of life' must yield to 'self-determination'.

Lord Goff re-asserted the illegality of active euthanasia, but said the turning off of a ventilator would be an omission rather than an act – so was therefore acceptable. This raised the question of whether or not withdrawing hydration and nutrition was sufficiently similar to withdrawing ventilation for it to also qualify as legally permissible withdrawal of care. Lord Goff thought that it was.

He also re-asserted it is only lawful to treat incompetent adults in their *best interests* (as per *F v. West Berkshire Health Authority*) and that in the Bland case 'the question is not whether it is in the best interests of the patient that he should die. The question is whether it is in his best interests that his life be prolonged by the continuance of this form of medical treatment or care.'

It was decided that termination of care should be carried out if treatment was *futile*. Lord Goff thought that questions of withdrawal of care should be subject to the *Bolam Test* (that is, would a reasonable body of medical practitioners act in a similar way?); however, he also thought that all similar cases involving the withholding of life-saving treatments should be brought before the courts.

Lord Mustill used slightly different reasoning. He also used *F v. West Berkshire Health Authority*, but said that Tony Bland, and other patients in PVS, have NO best interests as they are irreversibly unconscious, thus it is neither in his best interests to maintain treatment nor to withdraw it.

Key points of the Bland case were as follows:
- This case confirmed the *act/omission distinction* (see below).
- Withdrawal of treatment is not a culpable omission *if in the patient's best interests*.
- The case was decided on 'futility' of care, although some would argue feeding is not futile.

Moral conflicts in euthanasia
Acts and omissions
The act/omission debate centres on the question of whether actions are more culpable than omissions. In the euthanasia debate the question is whether there is a moral difference between killing someone (actively) and allowing them to die (passively) where their death is avoidable. The distinction between

killing someone and allowing someone to die is maintained in English Law.

The reasons for maintaining the act–omission distinction are that:

- Intuitively there seems to be a difference between killing and allowing to die.
- We make omissions all the time; for example, by *not* giving £50 per month to Oxfam I may allow the deaths of five people overseas, yet this does not seem as bad as actively killing five people.
- In practice the courts are easily able to distinguish acts from omissions, and find it useful to do so.

The reasons for ignoring the act–omission distinction are that:

- To the consequentialist, it does not matter whether the death was brought about by an act or an omission: both are choices we make and are ultimately responsible for.
- Some omissions can be relabelled quite easily as acts and vice versa. For example, is switching off a ventilator an act or an omission? If carried out by a patient's relative, it would be an act (and the relative could be charged with murder). If carried out by a doctor, it is seen as an omission.

Doctrine of double effect

As mentioned above, this doctrine was first mentioned in English Law in *R v. Bodkin Adams*. This doctrine, in essence, claims that it is sometimes morally permissible to carry out an action that has bad consequences which are foreseen but not intended. In the case of euthanasia this means that doctors may give strong painkillers to alleviate pain (intended consequence) even though such medication may shorten life (foreseen, but unintended consequence).

The doctrine holds if, and only if, four conditions are met (Hope et al. 2003):

1. The action (e.g. relieving pain) is good in itself.
2. The intention is solely to produce the good effect (i.e. the intent is to relieve pain, not to kill the patient).
3. The good effect is not achieved by the bad effect (i.e. killing the patient isn't the method by which the pain is relieved – it is a side effect of giving the pain medication).
4. There is sufficient reason to permit the bad effect (i.e. the relief of pain – that is the increase in quality of life – justifies the reduction in quantity of life).

There are a number of criticisms of this doctrine put forward by Glover (1977). The doctrine has a *distinction without a difference*. This is a criticism often levied by utilitarians who claim that the doctrine of double effect creates a distinction between foreseen and unintended consequences in scenarios where the outcomes are without difference. For example, if a pregnant woman with carcinoma of the uterus required the surgical removal of the uterus to save her life, with the foreseen but not intended death of the fetus, the doctrine would find this morally permissible. However, if treatment involved the direct killing of the fetus, this would not be acceptable, even though the consequences (death of the fetus and life-saving treatment of the mother) would be the same.

The doctrine also suffers the *problem of clarity*. Acts can be described in different ways according to one's viewpoint. For example, a suicide bombing on a bus may be described as making a political protest or as killing a busload of innocent people. Furthermore, it is unclear as to whether the deaths of the people on the bus are *intended* or merely *foreseen* consequences.

Arguments for euthanasia (adapted from Hope et al. 2003)
Consistency

- Suicide is accepted: it is commonly held that it is possible to rationally decide to kill oneself. Why then, should those who are unable to physically kill themselves be denied the right to choose how and when they should die, if in their opinion their life is no longer worth living? Perversely, it is the most disabled and ill who are least able to end their own lives. Do these people not deserve assistance if they wish to die?
- From passive to active euthanasia: the law currently allows the withdrawal and withholding of life-saving medical treatment. In the case of withholding nutrition (as in the Tony Bland case) death comes about due to dehydration and may take days or weeks to occur. If this kind of death is morally permissible, why should we not also permit active euthanasia, which by common intuition would seem to cause less suffering?
- From painkillers to lethal injections: if we allow the giving of painkillers that shorten life as well as relieving pain, and are unconvinced by the doctrine of double effect (see above), then why should we not give drugs that simply shorten life?

Appeal to principles

- Autonomy: respect for autonomy should mean assisting patients in bringing about their death when they so request.
- Beneficence: euthanasia is often described as 'mercy' killing. Death is seen as preferable to continued life with a high degree of suffering.

Arguments against euthanasia (adapted from Hope et al. 2003)

Improvements in palliative care mean euthanasia is unnecessary

- It is argued that palliative care is adequate to prevent suffering, and if the major argument for euthanasia is the reduction of suffering, the need for it is obviated.

Exploitation by others

- It is thought that some elderly or disabled people would consider themselves to be a burden on their family and carers, and whilst they may personally prefer to continue living, would request euthanasia in order to relieve their carers. It is also suggested that some people would be encouraged to request euthanasia by their families.

Slippery-slope objections

- If we allow euthanasia for the terminally ill, what then of people who are simply depressed or 'tired of living': would we also allow them to be euthanized? What about those with severe learning difficulties?

Contrary to the aims of medicine

- Some health-care professionals are opposed to euthanasia on the grounds that it is not what they consider to be part of the aims of medicine. In their view, health care is about prolonging life and reducing suffering, not causing death. Furthermore, patients may not trust their doctors if part of their role is carrying out euthanasia.

Death: when does 'death' occur (in collaboration with B. Ashmore)

In the past, death was accepted as an empirical matter and – as most dictionaries still define it – it is the end of life, the ceasing to be. However, technological advances have blurred the boundary of life and death. Some of the suggestions for the point at which death occurs are represented below.

In 1740 Jacques Winslow suggested that putrefaction was the only sure sign of death; here he implies *'death of the whole organism'*, and is suggesting that death involves every single cell ceasing to function and decomposing.

Cardio-respiratory arrest (i.e. the cessation of breathing and loss of a pulse) was the traditional indicator of death. However, it is no longer sufficient, as loss of consciousness, respiration, heartbeat, circulation and failure of the vital systems are no longer necessarily simultaneous events.

The concept of brain death emerged in France in 1959 when Mollaret and Goulon coined the phrase *Coma Dépassé* (a state beyond coma). The condition described as Coma Dépassé achieved worldwide recognition in 1968 under the guise of 'The Harvard Criteria', a protocol for defining brain death. It included four major criteria for 'brain death':

1. Absence of cerebral responsiveness.
2. Absence of induced or spontaneous movement.
3. Absence of spontaneous respiration.
4. Absence of brainstem and deep tendon reflexes.

Hypothermia and drug intoxication must be ruled out as differential diagnoses, and the tests must be repeated over 24 h. No patient meeting the Harvard Criteria has ever recovered, despite the most heroic management. It should be noted that in the UK 'brain death' is used to describe the destruction of the brainstem only (the concept 'brainstem death'). In the USA the term 'brain death' infers that the neocortex has also been destroyed (the concept of 'whole brain death').

Brainstem death (the UK version of brain death) is a compromise between two views:

1. That a person (or 'self') ceases to exist when they irreversibly lose the capacity for consciousness.
2. The human *organism* dies *only* when it ceases to function in an integrated way (biological death).

Death and the law in the UK

There is no statutory definition of death in English Law. Today, the medical profession's governing body has formally accepted that death is brainstem death.

Diagnosis of Brain Death (Anonymous 1976):

> It is agreed that the functional death of the brainstem constitutes Brain Death . . . it is good medical practice to recognize when Brain Death has occurred and act accordingly, sparing relatives from the further trauma of sterile hope.

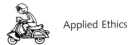

Diagnosis of Brain Death (Anonymous 1979):

It is the conclusion of the conference that the identification of Brain Death means that the patient is dead, whether or not the function of some organs, such as heartbeat, is maintained by artificial means.

There have been only two cases where the legality of such a position has been tested; both cases held that death had occurred at the point when the patient was pronounced brain dead. In a third case, this approach received the support of the House of Lords in *Airedale NHS Trust v. Bland*.

The Criminal Law Revision Committee considered the possibilities of drafting a new statute regarding brain death: 'If a statutory definition of death were to be enacted, there would, in our opinion, be a risk of further knowledge that would cause it to lose the assent of the majority of the medical profession. In that event, far from assisting the medical profession, for example, in the case of organ transplants, the definition may be a hindrance to them.' In essence, they claimed that a statute would be tantamount to fixing a medical opinion (which would take a long time to amend by due legal process), when such views rapidly evolve in the light of new evidence.

Is brain death a sufficient condition for defining death?

McCullagh summarized the reasons for thinking of the brain as the organ critical to identifying the death of the individual. They are:

- After irreversible cessation of brain function, all other organ systems will inevitably cease to function.
- Unlike other organ systems, brain function, once lost, is irreplaceable.
- Irreversible loss of brain function is synonymous with permanent loss of consciousness.
- Loss of sentience is a feature of loss of brain function.
- The integrative function of the brain is lost if the brain ceases to function.
- Death on the basis of loss of brain function is doing no more than recognizing overtly the reason underlying the traditional diagnosis of death following cessation of the blood circulation.
- If a patient is brain dead, but their body is maintained on an artificial ventilator, the cardiovascular, gastrointestinal and urinary systems continue to function. The body is warm,

consumes oxygen, and has a pulse. This is not a 'dead body', even if the patient is categorized as dead. The patient as a *person* is dead, but the body in some very important senses is alive. A brain-dead, ventilated body is still recognized as a living organism.

It is necessary to recognize that the concept of Brain Death does not represent a new way of being dead . . . there is only one way of being dead, and that is when the brain is dead. Tests for spontaneous cessation of cardio-respiratory functions are consequently only predictive of death. They amount to a necessary, but not sufficient, indicator of death.
(Lamb 1985)

Diagnosing death in a patient
As a house officer, you will be expected to certify the deaths of patients. The following is a guideline of what to do when a patient dies (Donald & Stein 2002):

1. See the body.
2. Confirm death:
   a. fixed and dilated pupils
   b. no respiratory effort – listen for three minutes
   c. no pulse or heart sounds for one minute.
3. If unsure, do an ECG.
4. Write in notes: 'Called to confirm death. No vital signs.'
5. Note the date and time of confirmation of death.
6. Sign and write your name clearly with your bleep number in the notes.
7. If possible, write down the cause(s) of death.
8. Note if the patient has a pacemaker or a radioactive implant.
9. Liaise with nurses about calling next of kin.
10. Inform GP.
11. Ask a senior if a post-mortem is desired and what cause(s) of death should be written on the death certificate.

Organ transplantation

Transplants are often seen as expensive, heroic experiments, rather than life-saving or life-improving procedures; it is perceived that they drain resources from routine and more cost-effective treatments. However:

- Kidney transplants were quoted as costing £4710 whereas hospital/home haemodialysis costs an *extra* £21 970/£17 260 (respectively).
- A heart transplant costing £7840 may be the only recourse to save a patient's life, whereas to remove a malignant tumour from the brain (which is a regularly performed life-saving intervention) would cost £107 780.

Although these measures are relatively crude, they show that transplantation compares well with other interventions that NHS resources already cover.

The shortage

At the end of December 1999, a total of 6676 patients were on the waiting lists in the UK (an increase of 3% on the previous year). Several thousand more who could benefit were not even on the waiting list. This is because only those who are considered to have a 'reasonable chance' of receiving a transplant are put on the list.

Twenty-five to 30% of patients die on waiting lists before organs are found. That equates to about 1000 people dying per year due to the shortage of donor organs.

The most suitable cadaveric donors are brainstem-dead individuals who have died in intensive therapy units (ITU), who are younger than 35 years (40 for women), and who have no history of organic heart disease.

In the UK during 1989 and 1990, an audit (Gore et al. 1992) found that of 24 000 people dying in intensive care, 3200 had a possible diagnosis of brain death by conventional definition. However, only 37% of these went on to become organ donors. Some of the reasons given for the loss of potential donors included:

- Brainstem death tests were not carried out in 39% of the cases.
- Relatives refused in 27% of the cases.
- Relatives were not asked in 6% of the cases.

Willingness to receive

Eighty-six per cent of respondents to a survey reported that they would accept a transplant 'if they really needed one', and only a small minority (7%) replied that 'transplantation would not be considered for religious, moral or other reasons'.

Willingness to give

A number of surveys asked respondents about their willingness to donate *their own* organs and their findings were very consistent, with seven in ten people (70%) willing to donate, and only 14% against donating their own organs. This indicates a widespread willingness amongst the UK population to donate their organs after they die.

However:

- Only one in five people regularly carried a donor card in the early 1990s (shown consistently throughout the three surveys), and approximately 70% do not have a donor card. The OPCS survey showed that only 27% of people without a card at present would think about getting one in the future. This leaves a large section of people who claim to be in favour of organ donation, but are unwilling to act.
- The NHS central organ donor register was launched in October 1994, yet five years later less than 14% of the population had registered.

The law and organ transplantation

The legislation governing organs and tissues includes:

- The Human Tissue Act 1961 – governs consent to transplanted organs.
- The Human Organ Transplants Act 1989 – governs LIVE donation of organs between genetically related donors and prohibits the SALE of organs.
- The Anatomy Act 1984 – governs the donation of bodies for dissection.

Remember: a person has no legal right in common law to determine what happens to their body after death. A body, or part of it, cannot be the subject matter of ownership.

The Human Tissue Act 1961

It is legal to remove organs for transplantation if:

- The deceased gave express consent in writing during their lifetime, or orally to two witnesses during their last illness.

   or

- The person 'lawfully in possession of the body' may authorize transplantation if there is no recorded declaration by the deceased. This can occur only when 'having made such reasonable enquiry as may be practicable' he/she can be sure

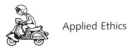
neither the deceased nor the 'surviving spouse, or any surviving relative' has any objection.

It should be noted that:
- The person 'lawfully in possession of the body' is usually the Hospital Authority – it is *not* the relatives.
- What 'reasonable enquiry' entails is vague and, technically, '*any*' surviving relative – however remote – can object to transplantation. As can a 'surviving' spouse, even if the couple has been separated for many years. In practice, hospitals usually seek the opinion only of those they consider to be 'close relatives'.
- There is no specific penalty for breach of this statute, and the Law Commission has held that had parliament intended to create an offence it would have done so expressly. However, health-care professionals are most likely to be sanctioned by the GMC for professional misconduct should they breach this statute.

The Human Organ Transplants Act 1989
This Act holds that organ transplants from a living person are illegal unless the person is genetically related to the recipient, OR they are referred through the Unrelated Live Transplant Regulatory Authority (ULTRA), which is an authority created by the Act to govern donation of organs between unrelated individuals.

Genetically related individuals include:
- Natural parents/children.
- Siblings (whole or half-blood relation).
- Aunts, uncles/nephews, nieces (whole or half-blood relation).

The definition of 'organ' is limited so as not to include replaceable tissues/fluids such as blood and plasma.

ULTRA transplants are governed by the *Human Organ Transplants (unrelated persons) Regulations (1989) SI 1989 No. 2480*. This seeks to ensure that:
- No payment has been made.
- The nature and risk of the procedure is explained to the donor.
- The donor is free from coercion.
- The donor has made fully informed consent.
- The donor is aware they can withdraw consent at any time.

It should be noted that:
- It is not possible to consent to the removal of an organ where death would become inevitable; so you cannot donate your heart or all of your liver.

- Patients who are incompetent can still donate, as long as it is in their *best interests*. For example, if they have a close emotional bond to the recipient.
- Whether children could ever donate more than bone marrow or blood seems unlikely, unless it too was clearly in their best interests.

The Human Tissue Act 2004 obtained Royal Assent in November 2004. This Act repeals the Human Tissue Act 1961, The Anatomy Act 1984 and The Human Organ Transplants Act 1989:
- The Act was produced in the wake of the Alder Hey Inquiry, and as a result places heavy emphasis on the importance of 'appropriate' consent when storing or utilizing tissue samples.
- The Act provides for the institution of the 'Human Tissue Authority', a regulatory body charged with the responsibility of inspecting and licensing those organizations involved in the storage and use of human tissue.
- The Act specifies criminal punishments for those acting outside the legislation.
- The Act prohibits the sale of any human material thereby making an organ market illegal.
- The Act does not affect the rights of coroners to demand a post-mortem and retain tissue without consent if they deem it necessary.

The ethics of organ transplantation
The field of organ transplantation raises a huge number of ethical questions. One way of thinking about the ethical dilemmas raised is by considering the problems caused by:
- Cadaveric organ donation.
- Organ donation from living people.
- Xenotransplantation.
- Methods of increasing organ supply.
- Resource allocation.

Cadaveric organ donation

There are ethical questions about the *definition of death*. Should the point of death be brainstem death or death of the entire brain cortex? Should we be allowed to keep brain-dead patients indefinitely ventilated if there is no need for their organs at the time of their death or to use them as self-replenishing blood banks? Should we choose to intubate dying patients in order to ventilate them when they die – even if it is of no benefit to them?

Organ donation from living people

The Human Organ Transplants Act was strict with regards to unrelated donations – perhaps because it assumed that altruistic donation is less likely between unrelated individuals. However, it seems plausible that family members may be under significant pressure to volunteer to donate an organ to an ailing relative. Children in particular may be pressured into donating to an ailing sibling.

Xenotransplantation

This is the transplantation of organs from animals to humans. Disadvantages of xenotransplantation may include:

- The cost of producing sterile transgenic animals (probably pigs) – which will have to be researched, tested and pass stringent safety requirements. Research questions will include:
  - whether it is appropriate to spend limited resources researching this technology when there are other methods to increase organ supply – such as an 'opt-out' system (see below)
  - whether the risk of introducing animal pathogens into the human population is justified.
- The ethics of treating animals as disposable commodities in this manner – raising animals simply as a source of spare organs. However, the widespread acceptance of factory farming and other livestock practices demonstrates a readiness to treat animals as commodities (although this is not necessarily an ethically justifiable position).

Methods of increasing organ supply

There are a number of different propositions for increasing organ supply. These include:

- *Mandated choice* – one of the problems with the current system (an 'opt-in' system) is that often no-one knows how the donor would have felt in life about donating organs, so relatives are consulted at a time when they are newly bereaved. The mandated choice would force citizens to answer whether or not they wish to donate their organs after death; this choice would be held on a central register and then held to be binding in the event of their organs being suitable for donation. People could be asked when registering with a GP, or via electoral registration.
- *Presumed consent* (an 'opt-out' system) – this system would not require everyone to be asked, rather it would assume that organs will be available for donation after death, unless individuals had registered the choice *not* to donate organs after death. At the moment, the wishes that the deceased had expressed in life are usually subordinate to those of the relatives.
- *Organ markets* – there are a number of ways this might work. Money could be paid to living donors – to donate kidneys for example. Or certain rewards could be given to the families who agree to the donation of organs from their relatives, for example help with funeral expenses. Utilitarian arguments would support an organ market if it led to more lives being saved at a reduced cost; such a system might well benefit donors (or their families) and those in need of treatment. However, arguments against this method include:
  - it is contrary to human dignity to commodify the human body by allowing the sale of organs
  - it would lead to exploitation of the poor by coercing the least well-off to sell their body parts.

Resource allocation

Given that there is a shortage of organs, and that patients die whose lives could feasibly be saved, is it fair that the relatives of potential donors can prevent viable organs being distributed to such patients? There has traditionally been more concern for the grieving process of the newly bereaved rather than for the need of those on the organ waiting list. Yet if we weigh the interest of the relatives (in not having organs removed from their loved one) against that of patients who need organ transplants *in order to remain alive*, we are hard-pressed to justify being in favour of the relatives.

Given that there is a shortage of organs, who should get priority in receiving a transplant? Currently, children receive organs in preference to adults. So a 16-year-old will receive a new kidney in preference to a 19-year-old. However, a 19-year-old won't be treated in preference to a 59-year-old – isn't this inconsistent?

- Outline five views on the moral worth of the human embryo.
- What are the circumstances in which an abortion can be carried out?
- Outline the pro-life v. pro-choice debate.
- What is the HFEA?
- What are the flaws in the '*it's unnatural*' argument?
- What does the Children Act 1989 say about the welfare of the child?
- What is Fraser competence?
- What justification is there for the compulsory detention of the mentally ill?
- What is the purpose of Section 2 of the Mental Health Act?
- What is the purpose of Section 3 of the Mental Health Act?
- What is the difference between voluntary, non-voluntary and involuntary euthanasia?
- What is the *doctrine of double effect*?
- What is the difference between an act and an omission?
- When is the DNAR acceptable?
- Which statutes govern the use of cadaveric organs, organs from living donors and body parts for dissection?
- Name three ways of increasing organ supply.

References

Amarakone K, Capps B Is it time to stop cloning about? Unpublished

Anonymous 1976 Diagnosis of brain death. Statement issued by the honorary secretary of the conference of Medical Royal Colleges and their Faculties in the United Kingdom on 11 October 1976. British Medical Bulletin 2(6045): 1187–8

Anonymous 1979 Diagnosis of brain death. Memorandum issued by the honorary secretary of the conference of Medical Royal Colleges and their Faculties in the United Kingdom on 15 January 1979. British Medical Bulletin 1(6159): 332

Donald A, Stein M 2002 The Hands-on Guide for House Officers, 2nd edn. Oxford: Blackwell Publishing, p. 94

Glover J 1977 Causing Death and Saving Lives. Harmondsworth: Pelican Books, Ch. 6

Gore SM, Cable DJ, Holland AJ 1992 Organ donation from intensive care units in England and Wales: two year confidential audit of deaths in intensive care. British Medical Journal 304 (6823): 349–55

Harris J 1994 The Value of Life. London: Routledge

Hoggett B 1996 Mental Health Law, 4th edn. London: Sweet & Maxwell, p. 32

Hope T, Savulescu J, Hendrick J 2003 Medical Ethics and Law. Edinburgh: Churchill Livingstone

Lamb D 1985 Death, Brain Death and Ethics. Albany, NY: State University of New York Press

McCullagh P 1993 Brain Dead, Brain Absent, Brain Donors. Chichester: John Wiley & Sons Ltd

McHale J, Fox M, Murphy J 1997 Health Care Law: texts and materials. London: Sweet & Maxwell, p. 373

Peele R, Chodoff P 1999 The ethics of involuntary treatment and deinstitutionalization. In Bloch S, Chodoff P, Green SA (eds) Psychiatric Ethics, 3rd edn. Oxford: Oxford University Press, pp. 430–1

Further reading

Bloch S, Chodoff P, Green SA (eds) 1999 Psychiatric Ethics, 3rd edn. Oxford: Oxford University Press

Brazier M 1992 Medicine, Patients and the Law, 2nd edn. Harmondsworth: Penguin

Harris J (ed.) 2001 Bioethics. Oxford: Oxford University Press

Harris J, Holm S (eds) 1998 The Future of Human Reproduction. Oxford: Oxford University Press

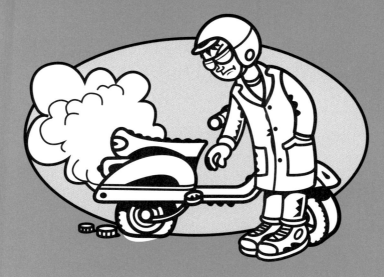

SOCIOLOGY AND PUBLIC HEALTH

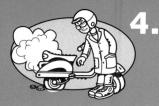

4. Sociology and Public Health Medicine

Why is sociology important to medical students?

Sociology has been one of the latest additions to the medical student's curriculum. Its importance lies in its ability to explain health and disease using a perspective different from that of the standard biomedical model.

Arguably, the role of health-care professionals is to provide holistic care – that is caring for the *whole person*; therefore, medical students ought to be learning how to accomplish this. Sociology is about '*understanding the individual's place in the world*: where they are, what they do and what their views are' (Iphofen & Poland 1998). The key points of sociology include the following:

- Sociology is a *scientific* discipline.
- Sociology aims to take an *objective* look at ordinary behaviour as well as abnormal behaviour.
- Sociology deals with both *quantitative* and *qualitative* data.
- Within the medical field sociology is concerned with causes, prevention and treatment of disease; the effect of disease on patients, their families and society in general; how patients and health-care professionals interact; and the role of medicine in society. Furthermore, a little reading and understanding of core concepts in sociology can go a long way in an exam!

Important areas that need to be covered before your exams:
- Basic definitions.
- The biological vs. holistic model of health.
- The changing pattern of disease.
- Social causes of disease.
- Different ways of measuring the health of the nation.

Epidemiology

Epidemiology is the study of the distribution and the determinants of health or ill-health in whole populations, and its application to modify this distribution. In other words, epidemiologists are concerned with the health of the whole population as opposed to the health of the individual patient.

Epidemiology is the study of 'how' and 'why' diseases occur in a population.

Public health is the systematic application of epidemiology, i.e. the promotion of health and disease prevention, thus prolonging life and improving the quality of life through the concerted efforts of society.

Since the 1960s, epidemiology has become important in assessing risk factors for, and reducing the incidence of, multi-factorial diseases such as heart disease.

Epidemiological approach:
- Definition of disease.
- Aetiology or cause of disease.
- How disease spreads/occurs – the risk factors in individuals both within the population and in the environment.
- How to control disease.
- How to prevent disease.
- How to eliminate disease.

There are a myriad uses for this discipline in planning health-care provision.
These include:
- Identifying factors that can affect the occurrence of disease.
- Assessing the effectiveness of preventive and therapeutic treatments (this is sometimes known as *clinical epidemiology*).
- Assessing the impact of health-care services.
- Predicting future health-care needs.

Until 1968, smallpox disease killed 10 million people worldwide per year. The eradication of this disease in 1979 was heralded as the single greatest achievement of the public health initiatives (Fig. 4.1).

Smallpox eradication plan	
STEP	**ANSWER**
Definition	Infectious disease
Cause	*Variola* virus
Risk factors	Overcrowding, excessive mobility of population due to political instability and extreme poverty leading to poor hygiene and poor nutrition
Control	Risk factors could not be altered adequately, so decided to eliminate virus
Prevention	Administer smallpox vaccine en masse. Also continuous surveillance and containment of infected patients

Fig. 4.1 Smallpox eradication plan, illustrating the epidemiological approach.

Measures of disease occurrence

Two basic measurements are used to assess the frequency of ill-health events: incidence and prevalence (Figs 4.2, 4.3).

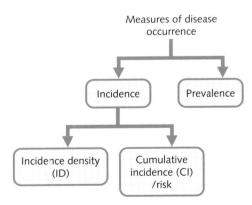

Fig. 4.2 Measures of disease occurrence.

Incidence

Incidence quantifies the number of **new** cases of a disease within a specified time-interval. It measures a change from a healthy state to a diseased state. Hence it can only be assessed using follow-up studies e.g.

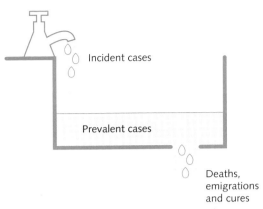

Fig. 4.3 Characteristics of incidence and prevalence.

cohort-studies. There are two categories of incidence rate: cumulative incidence and incidence density.

Cumulative incidence

Cumulative incidence (CI) is the proportion of unaffected individuals who, on average, will contract the disease in question over a period of time.

$$CI = \frac{A \text{ (no. of new cases of disease in a given period of time)}}{N \text{ (no. of disease-free persons at the beginning of that period of time)}}$$

Incidence density

Cumulative incidence assumes that the entire population at risk at the beginning of the study has been followed up for the *entire* specified period of time. Often, however, some participants will enter the study years after the start, and some will be lost to follow-up before the study ends. This is a *dynamic* population. In these circumstances, the length of follow-up will not be uniform for all participants.

Incidence density (ID) accounts for these varying time-periods of follow-up and the denominator can be calculated to represent the sum of the individuals' times at risk, i.e. the sum of time that each person remained under observation and was at risk. This is called the *person-time* (PT):

$$PT = \text{average size of population at risk} \times \text{average length of observation}$$

The ID measures the rapidity with which newly diagnosed cases of the disease develop:

$$ID = \frac{A}{PT}$$

Prevalence

This indicates the number of existing cases of the disease of interest in a population. As it is often measured at a particular point in time, it is called *point prevalence*(P).

$$P = \frac{C \text{ (no. of cases in a defined population at one point in time)}}{N \text{ (no. of persons in a defined population of the same size)}}$$

Prevalence is a proportion. It is the only measure of disease occurrence that can be obtained from *cross-sectional studies*. It measures the burden of disease, i.e. the status of a condition in the population.

The changing pattern of disease

As populations change, the pattern of prevalent disease within it also changes. This is evident in England from the changing pattern of disease over time, as reflected in mortality rates and life expectancy at birth (Gray 2001):

- In 1851 mortality in England: 22.7 per 1000 population.
- In 2001 mortality in England: 11.9 per 1000 population.
- In 1901 life expectancy: men – 47 years; women – 50 years.
- In 2001 life expectancy: men – 75 years; women – 80 years.

These figures show that average life expectancy has been increased by around 30 years in the past century. This has been achieved in the main by the reduction of *infant* and *child* mortality. The average life expectancy of a 50-year-old individual in 1850 and a 50-year-old today has not greatly increased.

Life expectancy helps us to assess the health status of a population. It is defined as the average number of years one can expect an individual of a given age to live if current mortality trends continue.

The mortality rates and life expectancies that the UK experienced 150 years ago are similar to current rates of developing world countries: (e.g. Ethiopia – mortality of 23.6 per 1000).

The changing pattern of disease and society

As different types of society have evolved, the major causes of disease have changed.

Pre-agricultural society

Little is known about the health and risks to health of pre-agricultural societies. It is assumed that the major health risks were environmental.

Agricultural society

Agricultural societies produced the bulk of their food by growing crops and through the domestication of animals. As the lifestyle was no longer nomadic, the populations were of a greater density and sanitation was poor. As a result air-borne (TB), water-borne (cholera), food-borne (dysentery) and vector-borne (malaria) infectious diseases become the major health risk.

Modern industrial societies

Infectious disease has become gradually less important in modern societies. This is probably due to:

- Decreased exposure to pathogens, due to changes in domestic housing and reduction in contamination of food and water supplies.
- Improved nutrition, especially in mothers and children.
- Increased acquired resistance to infection and the ability to recover from infection – due to improved nutrition.
- Specific medical intervention – for example, antibiotics and vaccinations.
- Economic development and improved standard of living.

However, some populations are still vulnerable to certain infections, e.g the elderly tend to get pneumonia and certain immigrant populations are at a higher risk of TB. In addition to this, certain infections are now becoming an increasing problem due to antibiotic resistance.

Major causes of death now include:
- Coronary heart disease.
- Cancers.
- Respiratory disease.
- Strokes.

Major causes of morbidity include:
- Arthritis.
- Obesity and diabetes.
- Mental-health problems.

The Government's health strategy as laid out in *Saving Lives: Our Healthier Nation* (Department of Health, 1999) identifies the following four main targets:

- *Coronary heart disease* – 40% cut in death rate in under 75s between 1997 and 2010.
- *Cancer* – 20% cut in death rate in under 75s between 1997 and 2010.
- *Mental Health* – 20% cut in death rate in under 75s between 1997 and 2010.
- *Accidents* – 20% cut in death rate in under 75s between 1997 and 2010.

'Developing world' diseases

The global pattern of disease varies greatly between 'developed' and 'developing' countries. The developed world has a greater burden of non-communicable degenerative disease, e.g. cardiovascular disease, stroke, respiratory disease, cancers and mental illness. In the developing world, the main causes of death are also cardiovascular, stroke and respiratory disease. In addition communicable or infectious diseases, e.g. malaria, TB and HIV/AIDS, are major killers and causes of ill-health in the population. The younger population tends to suffer more. About 70% of young children who die from diarrhoeal diseases could be saved if widespread low-cost oral rehydration therapy was available. The problem is compounded by the lack of adequate sanitation, clean water and nutrition; these are commonly exacerbated in conflict zones. Malaria can easily be prevented by prophylactic measures, e.g. sleeping under mosquito nets, but the cost of implementing these is great. There is also an emerging resistance to the drugs normally used to treat malaria.

The solution to these problems will take roughly the same route as that taken by developed countries. Possible areas of intervention include trying to improve national and local wealth, living standards, clean water supplies and sanitation, nutrition and educational status of the people, particularly the women. A greater commitment and degree of transparency is also required by the respective governments (Fig. 4.4).

Social causes of disease

Western medicine has been based upon what is known as the *biomedical model*. This makes the following assumptions:

1. The mind and body can be treated separately – *mind–body dualism*.
2. The body can be treated as a machine – *the mechanical metaphor*.
3. Technological interventions are generally successful in the treatment of disease – *the technological imperative*.
4. Explanations of disease focus on biological changes rather than social and psychological factors – that is, they are *reductionist* in nature.
5. Reductionist explanations have led to the *doctrine of specific aetiology* – where it is assumed that every disease is caused by a specific identifiable agent or 'disease entity' (see below).

The success of the biomedical model has been, in part, attributed to its claim that it is an *objective* science – with a gradual increase in the truth of explanations provided. Medicine has, thus, claimed to be the only valid response to the understanding of disease and illness. Sociology has sought causes of disease beyond the reductionistic – or simply biological – level (Fig. 4.5).

What is a 'cause' of disease?

A cause is generally understood to be the one thing that brings about a change in another. For example

Fig. 4.4 Factors affecting health.

Factors affecting health				
Fixed	**Social and economic**	**Environment**	**Lifestyle**	**Access to services**
Genes	Poverty	Air quality	Diet	Education
Sex	Employment	Housing	Physical activity	NHS
Ageing	Social exclusion	Water quality	Smoking	Social services
		Social environment	Alcohol	Transport
			Sexual behaviour	Leisure
			Drugs	

Source: adapted from Nettleton S 1995 The Sociology of Health and Illness. Cambridge: Polity Press, pp. 5–6

Fig. 4.5 Challenges to the biomedical model.

Challenges to the biomedical model
The efficacy of the biomedical model has been exaggerated
The reduction in disease in the Western world has more to do with improved social conditions, i.e. sanitation, housing, availability of fresh food, etc., than with medical advances such as vaccinations and antibiotics
The causes of disease are multi-factorial
Focusing on the biological changes has underestimated the links between material circumstances and illness. An underappreciation of the social factors may have led to a failure to account for the inequalities of health
Biomedicine has failed to account for socio-cultural interpretations of disease that influence an individual's perception and experience of health and illness
Sociologists have suggested that some disease is *socially constructed*, and, therefore, by attempting to examine only the biological dysfunction, biomedical models miss much of the cause and, therefore, potential cure. Even apparently biologically based disease may be directly brought about by social factors

Source: adapted from Nettleton S 1995 The Sociology of Health and Illness. Cambridge: Polity Press, pp. 5–6

we can say atheroma causes ischaemic heart disease. This is a 'monocausal' model. It can be written as:

A → B: where A is the cause and B is the effect

Of course, the causality of ischaemic heart disease is more complicated than atheroma – because this simple model begs the questions 'What causes atheroma?' and 'How does atheroma cause ischaemic heart disease?' Atheroma can be increased or decreased by promoting or inhibiting factors. A multicausal model is more appropriate. Factors such as genetic predisposition, poverty, poor diet, smoking, diabetes, oral contraceptives may be promoting factors, whereas physical activity, access to medical health care and polyunsaturated fats may be inhibitors. The possible multicausal model is illustrated in Figure 4.6.

In order to establish a cause there are three conditions that need to be fulfilled:

1. Temporal sequence – the cause must precede the effect – if it does not, the relationship cannot be causal.

2. Correlation between cause and effect – the effect should vary with the cause – so increased atheroma should lead to increased incidence of ischaemic heart disease.

3. There should be no third variable. For example, cases of gout might increase with the number of cars owned. The third variable here might be increased affluence, which may lead to a richer diet or drinking more port, which may cause increased gout (Fig. 4.7).

Theories of disease causation
Germ theory
- Germ theory was established during the late 1800s, when scientists such as Ehrlich, Koch and Pasteur isolated various disease-causing organisms.

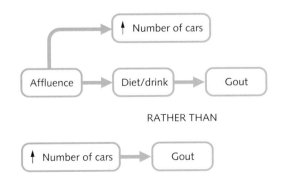

Fig. 4.7 The confusion that can result when a third variable is introduced.

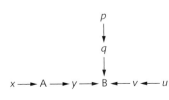

Fig. 4.6 A multicausal model for disease.

- Koch (who isolated the bacillus that causes TB) established the idea that a disease agent must always be found with the disease in question, rather than be found with other diseases.
- The purpose of medical practice was to identify these agents then neutralize them.
- This is a 'monocausal' model.

Epidemiological triangle
- This refined the 'germ theory'.
- Disease is seen as an interaction between three entities:
  – the host
  – the disease agent
  – the environment.
- Exposure to the disease agent is necessary for the disease to manifest – but not sufficient.
- The disease can be prevented by modifying factors that influence exposure and susceptibility. This is a 'multicausal' model.
- More useful in understanding causation of infectious diseases than chronic, degenerative ones.

Web of causation
- Disease results from the complex interaction of many risk factors.
- Any risk factor can be implicated in more than one disease.
- Disease can be prevented by modifying these risk factors.

General susceptibility
- This theory has grown out of the observation that certain groups (for example, the lower social classes or people who have been divorced) are more susceptible to a number of diseases (see Chapter 7).
- It is not concerned with the individual risk factors – rather the general susceptibility to disease and death.
- General susceptibility is probably a result of environment, lifestyle, behaviour and genetic predisposition.

(Adapted from Locker 2003, p. 20)

Socioenvironmental approach
- A refinement of the 'general susceptibility' theory.
- Recognizes social and physical environments have a heavy effect on health and disease.
- Identifies socioenvironmental risks, physiological risks, behavioural risk, and psychosocial risks.

- The interaction between the above types of risks affects health status.
- Suggests the importance of protective/vulnerability factors that help to explain why some people are less/more at risk than others.

(Adapted from Locker 2003)

Social structures and health
Social integration, support and life events The sociologist *Emile Durkheim* argued that industrialization had led to a loss of social integration, due to an emphasis on individualism, division of labour and specialization of tasks. He supposed that suicide could be explained in terms of how individuals were integrated into their social group and that suicide would be associated with very excessive or very deficient social integration. In industrialized societies where underintegration is a primary hazard, the greatest risk of suicide would be in those who were most isolated. He hypothesized that:

- Single people, widows and widowers should show a higher rate of suicide than similar, married individuals.
- Suicides would decrease in wartime when community spirit was more prevalent.
- Protestants, who were less well integrated into their religious community, would have a higher rate of suicide than Jews or Catholics.

Other studies have also shown the wider benefits to health of social support. Gove (1973) showed that the single, widowed and divorced had higher rates of mortality, and a number of diseases (Fig. 4.8).

There are a number of reasons why marital status might make an indirect difference to health:
- Married couples may be happier, or experience less stress, and are less likely to be socially isolated.
- Marriage might confer meaning upon the lives of individuals imbuing them with a sense of purpose.
- The trauma of separation or not being married may lead to risky behaviours such as smoking or drinking.
- The presence of a partner may encourage medical advice to be sought early on in disease.
- Single, never married, people may start off as less healthy – thereby failing to get married.

Other studies have looked into social support and its effect on health:

Marital status and mortality	Married	Single	Widowed	Divorced
Mortality	1.00	1.95	2.64	3.39
Lung cancer	1.00	1.45	2.24	3.07
Diabetes	1.00	2.69	2.46	4.32
Liver cirrhosis	1.00	3.29	4.61	8.84
Leukaemia	1.00	1.07	0.91	1.28

Source: Gove WR 1973

Fig. 4.8 Marital status and mortality.

- Social support was defined in terms of marital status, *number* of contacts with friends/relatives and membership of religious/social groups – to give a social network score.
- Low social network scores associated with increased risk of early mortality (two to three times above those with high network scores).
- Church attendance was related to low mortality scores (although a single component in a wider social network).
- Increased heart disease was shown with low social support.
- Increased complications in pregnancy were associated with low social support.
- Increased emotional illness was associated with low social support.
- A lack of social support, social isolation and being unmarried reduced men's life expectancy following an initial myocardial infarction.
- A higher risk of suicide was found in divorced men and was twice that of married men.

However, in a study of women and depression the following was found:
- Social support was protective in the context of a severe life event but was not so beneficial in other circumstances.

The lack of consistency and clarity of the findings may be due to the difficulties associated with accurate measurement of 'social support'. The relationship between social support and health may be due to the following factors:
- Increased provision of information about health.
- Increased psychological support.
- Support acts as a buffer against the negative effects of adverse life events (this suggests that social support is not beneficial in itself – rather it is protective against life problems).

Adverse life events The association between severe life events, such as bereavement, and illness, such as depression, led to the idea that life events may be important in the aetiology of a variety of diseases.

Holmes & Rahe (1967) developed the Social Readjustment Rating Scale (SRRS). This consisted of a number of life events that were given a score depending on how life changing each event was, for example:
- Death of wife/husband – 100.
- Divorce – 73.
- Marriage – 50.
- Retirement – 45.
- Moving house – 20.

A number of studies have shown a correlation between the score of a life event and adverse health consequences. Problems with this scale include:
- Life events can be of variable meaning to individuals – moving house may be a positive or a negative experience, as could retirement.
- The scale neglects minor, but perhaps more frequent or chronic problems.

Social and cultural change Some of the earliest social factors studied dealt with industrialization and the rural to urban migration of large populations. In Britain this happened during the industrial revolution. (A similar process is now happening in much of the developing world.) Prior to that time few families were entirely wage-dependent – rather, they worked the land tied to the home and exchanged produce for necessities. The industrial revolution transformed the workforce into large groupings of employees who were solely dependent on the wages they received. Subsistence became increasingly difficult – purchasing power became

73

dependent on employment. Aside from the changes in employment, migration has further effects on health and disease.

Geographical mobility encourages the spread of infectious diseases, but its effect on non-communicable diseases is less clear-cut. This may be because people migrate for different reasons, and this may affect the impact of mobility on morbidity. Armstrong (1989) outlines three reasons for movement between countries:

1. *Mass migration* – when all age groups in a population move. This may be due to war, famine or other disaster.
2. *Economic migration from an underdeveloped country* – often young unskilled men.
3. *Economic migration from a developed country* – tends to be professionals or skilled workers.

Migrants are thought to suffer from higher levels of depression, insomnia and anxiety. This may be explained by factors such as language difficulties, hostility in the host country, new cultural practices and so on. However, this level of illness associated with migration may be dependent on the reasons for migration (more illness in refugees than economic migrants) and the ability of the migrants to adopt local lifestyles – a process known as 'acculturation'.

In a study looking at the health of Japanese migrants in California compared with the health of Japanese people in Japan:

- Coronary heart disease was increased in the migrants.
- There was large variation within the migrants – with those continuing to follow traditional Japanese customs having lower heart disease.
- Coronary heart disease was increased in those who had adopted Western lifestyles.

Another study showed that the proportion of South Asians undergoing coronary artery revascularization was much lower than that of the Caucasian population, even though they suffer from more severe angina. In a UK study it was shown that Asian, West Indian and African immigrants as a whole had about twice the rate of British-born subjects of having a first admission to the hospital for mental illness.

From observations of women from ethnic minorities or from non-English-speaking backgrounds, another study concluded that these women should be regarded as a high-risk group for postnatal depression.

Measuring the health of the nation

Routine data are not often collected for a specific research purpose; however, such data may contain information associated with health and social services. Epidemiologists have access to a multitude of data sources. The accuracy, validity and completeness of such information depends on how regularly it is used and, hence, how much attention is paid to it (Figs 4.9, 4.10).

Some different sources of data are outlined below.

Demographic data

This provides us with the denominators necessary to calculate incidence and prevalence. The best example is the *census* that is conducted every ten years and gives details on family size, socio-economic status, highest level of education attained, and the age, sex distribution and geographical location of the population. The *GHS* (*General Household Survey*) collects data from a questionnaire administered to a stratified random sample of households. Data collected relates to population, employment, housing, education, income and family structure and details on many health-related items, such as prevalence of disability, utilization of general practitioners' services, dietary habits, alcohol and tobacco consumption.

Mortality data

This is based upon completion of a standard death certificate, which records the date of death, cause of death, age, sex, date of birth and place of residence. In addition, occupation and other variables may be recorded. Certain causes of death may be poorly recorded. In the UK, for example, it has been shown that deaths from HIV disease and AIDS, which may be stigmatized, are under-recorded in an attempt to maintain confidentiality. Other problems are that data from urban areas may be more complete than data from rural areas, and people belonging to higher social classes are likely to have a more detailed cause of death recorded. The main cause of death in an individual is that pathological process that directly led to the patient's death. The patient may have other co-morbid conditions that worsen the prognosis, but do not directly lead to death, e.g. diabetes or hypertension.

Fig. 4.9 Sources of routine data.

Sources of routine data	
Demographic and lifestyle data	Census General Household Survey (GHS) Registrar of births and marriages
Morbidity data	Morbidity statistics from general practice Communicable disease surveillance – infectious disease notification Hospital in-patient enquiry Hospital activity analysis/Hospital Episode System (HES) Cancer registration GP morbidity
Mortality data	Office for National Statistics (ONS) Mortality Statistics Registrar General's Decennial Supplement on Occupational Mortality
Specific datasets	ONS Survey of Disability ONS Longitudinal Study Abortion data Congenital anomalies Workmen's compensation data
Health service data	Immunization levels achieved Uptake of cervical cancer and breast cancer screening District and regional annual reports Chief Medical Officer's annual report Reviews of peri-operative mortality and maternal mortality
Other	Social security statistics Private sector and voluntary organization data

Pros and cons of routine data	
Value of routine data	Limitations of routine data
Readily available	Lack of completeness, with potential for bias – may not answer the question
Already collected and available	Incomplete ascertainment as not every case is captured
Standardized collection procedures	Limited details of determinants such as income and ethnicity
Limited costs	Often poorly presented and analyzed – need careful interpretation
Up to date and relatively comprehensive; available for past years	Disease labelling may vary over time, e.g. asthma definition has been changing
Wide range of recorded items	Coding changes may create artefactual ↑/↓ in rates
Experience in use and interpretation	Occasionally subject to political influences and manipulation
Useful for identifying hypotheses	Health services' data more geared to process than health status and outcomes
Useful for initial assessment	Large sample sizes
Provides baseline data on expected levels of health/disease	

Fig. 4.10 Pros and cons of routine data.

Morbidity data

Morbidity data are often routinely available and provide insights into conditions that may not necessarily result in death. Certain communicable diseases, e.g. meningitis, malaria, need to be reported by law. This information is sent to the Public Health Laboratory Service who surveys and monitors the reported incidence of communicable diseases and detects unusual patterns or epidemics.

Death certification

The process of death certification in England and Wales is currently under review, and is likely to be overhauled following the Harold Shipman case and a general dissatisfaction with the way in which deaths are certified by doctors.

Studies of the accuracy of death certification have found up to one-third of death certificates to contain major errors. A recent English study reported that only 55% of certificates were completed to an acceptable standard. The main explanations for these errors are:

- Lack of training of doctors.
- Inadequate or misunderstood clinical information.
- Concealment of information that might distress family member.
- Omissions of information.
- Coding errors.

Variations between countries in the post-mortem criteria may also lead to differences in diagnostic information and hence the cause of death.

The certificate of death registration (DC) is vital for the funeral to proceed. A doctor may complete this form only if he or she has been in attendance on the deceased during the last illness and has seen the deceased within 14 days of death or after death. There are some cases that have to be reported to the coroner:

- Violent deaths.
- Deaths when a doctor has not attended in the previous 14 days.

 There are three categories of death: those certified by a doctor, those certified by a doctor with the coroner's agreement and those reported to and investigated by the coroner.

- When the cause of death is unknown or uncertain.
- Accidental death.
- Doubtful stillbirth.
- Deaths related to surgery or anaesthetic.
- Deaths within 24 hours of admission to hospital.

When a death is reported to the coroner he may: certify the death on the basis of the information he has or acquires; certify the death after ordering an autopsy; or certify the death after holding an inquest.

The DC must reach the coroner's office in five days (Fig. 4.11).

Scenario

Trevor Smith, a 65-year-old retired musician, is registered blind secondary to his diabetic retinopathy and so does not see the flight of steps. He tumbles down and is unable to move. He is discovered by a neighbour after two days. You are the house officer on call at the hospital. He has fractured the neck of his right femur and you are instructed to prepare him for theatre. Suddenly he becomes dyspnoeic and you see that the electrocardiograph (ECG) shows sinus tachycardia. His arterial blood gases suggest respiratory failure. A ventilation perfusion (V/Q) scan shows a V/Q mismatch. Three hours later he enters cardiorespiratory arrest. You start cardiopulmonary resuscitation and put out a crash call. After 25 minutes' resuscitation, he remains unresponsive and the crash team decides to stop.

Trevor Smith's death certificate

1.
   a. Pulmonary embolus (hours). You can justify this because of the ECG, blood gas results, and V/Q scan result. Note that uninvestigated shortness of breath three hours before death alone would be no good.
   b. Fat embolus (days). From his fractured neck of femur.
2. Insulin dependent diabetes mellitus (20 years).

Measures of health and treatment outcomes

Mortality rates

The simplest form of mortality measure is the *crude mortality rate* (CMR).

$$CMR = \frac{\text{No. of deaths in a specified period} \times 100}{\text{Average total population during that period}}$$

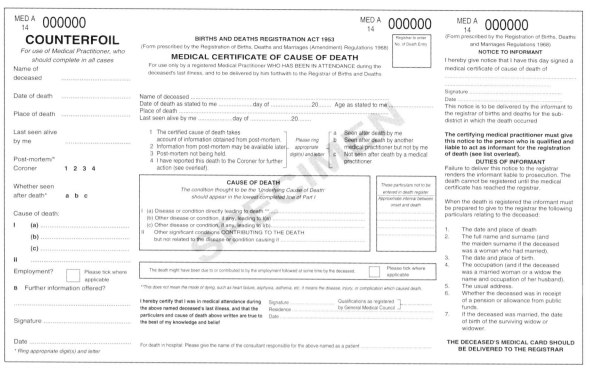

Fig. 4.11 Medical certification of cause of death.

The main advantage of using the CMR is that mortality can be expressed as a single figure. This is useful when comparing mortality within an area over a period of time. However, the main disadvantage is that it does not take into account that the chance of dying varies according to age and sex. In fact, standardization is usually aimed at age and sex alone because the effects of these are normally taken as given, whereas possible differences in relation to race and social class are issues for research.

Specific mortality rates refer to the number of deaths occurring in a sub-group of the population. To aid this, there are age-specific and gender-specific mortality rates. These help to detect which parts of the community are most affected by mortality.

$$\text{Age/sex-specific death rate} = \frac{\text{No. of deaths in each age/sex group in a period}}{\text{Average no. of people in age/sex population in a period}}$$

Standardized rates take into account the different age/sex structure of two populations so that their mortality experience can be compared directly. Hence, we eliminate the confounding factors of age and sex.

The most common means of comparison is the *standardized mortality ratio* (SMR), which is the ratio of observed deaths to expected deaths expressed as a percentage:

$$\text{SMR} = \frac{\text{Observed deaths} \times 100}{\text{Expected deaths}}$$

An SMR of 100 indicates that observed deaths equals the expected number of deaths (average mortality). An SMR >100 indicates observed deaths exceed expected deaths, and an SMR <100 indicates observed deaths lower than expected deaths.

It is worth noting that the process of standardizing mortality rates is a complex process. There are two methods of standardization, *indirect* and *direct*.

Potential years of life lost

- The potential years of life lost (PYLL) is an indicator of premature mortality. It represents the total number of years NOT lived by an individual who died before age 75 years.
- This indicator gives more importance to the causes of death that occurred at younger ages than those that occurred at older ages.
- The upper age limit of 75 years is used to approximate the life expectancy as that is

considered the average life-span for someone in good health.

- Deaths occurring in individuals aged 75 years or older are NOT included in the calculation.
- Infant deaths – deaths among infants under one year of age – are not included in the calculation due to their very small numbers. Other methods exclude these deaths since they are often due to causes that have different aetiology from deaths at later ages.

Quality adjusted life years

Quality adjusted life years (QALYs) is a single health state measure combining quantity and quality of life (see also pp. 32–33). It is a generic measure that sums years spent in different health states using weights (on a scale of 0 (dead) to 1 (perfectly healthy) for each health state). So, 5 years of perfect health = 5 QALYs; 2 years in a state measured as 0.5 of perfect health followed by 3 years of perfect health = 4 QALYs.

Advantages
- Large studies using QALYs have reliable and valid results.
- Used in cost utility analysis – which allows comparison between interventions that nominally differ in terms of outcomes.

Disadvantages
- Theoretical questions: can moral judgements be made scientific?

- Difficult to understand consequences when healthy.
- Calculation is dependent on *who* is asked – patient, doctor, and *how* they are asked.

Morbidity (illness) rates

While death is (generally) a certain and countable event, mortality rates do not tell us much about illness or health in a population. Morbidity, illness and health are, however, considerably more difficult to define, and hence to measure, than death. The following measures are commonly used.

Health service use measures
- Consultation rates, e.g. with GP.
- Referral rates, e.g. by GP.
- Hospital admission and discharge rates.

These suffer from the problem that access to healthcare providers affects rate of usage.

Illness self-report rates
- General Household Survey (GHS).
- Sickness–absence rates.
- Specific survey studies using a validated questionnaire.

Each of these has its own limitations in terms of coverage. For example, sickness–absence rates do not

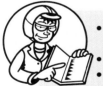

- Explain briefly the role of epidemiology and sociology in understanding the causes of disease.
- Justify the use of incidence and prevalence in showing the impact of a disease.
- Discuss the changing patterns of disease from the pre-agricultural era to modern-day living.
- Describe the socioeconomic impact of disease in the developing world.
- Briefly discuss the multifactorial models of disease.
- Compare and contrast the prevalence of diseases in the developing world with those in the developed world.
- Outline the effects of family, marriage and life events on an individual's health.
- Describe how social and cultural change has led to a change in the patterns of disease.
- Give an overview of the sources of data that epidemiologists use to measure the health of the nation.
- Highlight the different methods for measuring outcomes in health care.

include people who are not working, such as pensioners or the unemployed.

Despite being more difficult to measure, when used carefully morbidity rates can tell us much about ill-health in specific groups of the population.

References

Armstrong D 1989 An Outline of Sociology as Applied to Medicine, 3rd edn. London: Wright, p. 22

Department of Health 1999 Saving Lives: Our Healthier Nation Cm4386 London: HMSO. Available at http://www.archive.official-documents.co.uk/document/cm43/4386/4386.htm

Gove WR 1973 Sex, marital status and mortality. American Journal of Sociology 79: 45–67

Gray, A 2001 World Health and Disease, 3rd edn. Buckingham: Open University Press

Holmes TH, Rahe RH 1967 The social readjustment rating scale. Journal of Psychosomatic Research 213–18

Further reading

Berkman LF, Syme SL 1979 Social networks, host resistance, and mortality: a nine year follow-up study of Alameda County residents. American Journal of Epidemiology 109: 186–204

Carpenter L, Brockington IF 1980 A study of mental illness in Asians, West Indians and Africans living in Manchester. British Journal of Psychiatry 137: 201–5

Donaldson LJ, Donaldson RJ 2000 Essential Public Health, 2nd edn. Berkshire: Petroc Press

Feder G, Crook AM, Magee P, Banerjee S, Timmis AD, Hemingway H 2002 Ethnic differences in invasive management of coronary disease: prospective cohort study of patients undergoing angiography. BMJ 324(7336): 511–16

Fitzpatrick R 2003 Society and changing patterns of disease. In: Scambler G (ed.) Sociology as Applied to Medicine, 5th edn. Edinburgh: Saunders, pp. 3–17

Iphofen R, Poland F, Campling J 1998 Sociology in Practice for Health Care Professionals. Basingstoke: Palgrave

Locker D 2003 Social determinants of health and disease. In: Scambler G (ed.) Sociology as Applied to Medicine, 5th edn. Edinburgh: Saunders, pp. 18–33

McCormick A 1998 Trends in mortality statistics in England and Wales with particular reference to AIDS from 1984 to April 1987. British Medical Journal (Clinical Research Edition) 296 (6632): 1289–92

Marmot M, Syme L, Kagan A 1975 Epidemiological studies of heart disease and stroke in Japanese men living in Japan, Hawaii and California. Prevalence of coronary and hypertensive disease and associated risk factors. American Journal of Epidemiology 102: 514–25

Onozawa K, Kumar RC, Adams D, Dore C, Glover V 2003 High EPDS scores in women from ethnic minorities living in London. Archives of Women's Mental Health Aug (suppl 2): S51–5

Vetters N, Matthews I 1999 Environmental and occupational health-infectious disease. In: Vetters N, Matthews I. Epidemiology and Public Health Medicine. Edinburgh: Churchill Livingstone, pp. 129–36

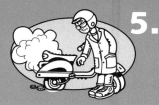

5. Experience of Health and Illness

Behaviour in health and illness

Illness behaviour and the sick role

In Chapter 4 we looked at how disease patterns have changed over time, and how social and environmental factors have played a causative role in the experience of disease. In this section we look at the processes that motivate individuals to utilize health services.

Hannay (1988) identifies five stages of illness:

1. The experience of symptoms (and illness behaviour).
2. Advice or consultation with friends/relatives – known as 'lay referral' (see p. 83).
3. Consultation with a doctor – to confirm subjective *illness* and gain objective diagnosis of *disease*. This stage *legitimizes* a *sick role*.
4. Being in the sick role as a dependent patient.
5. Recovery.

Each of these stages can be affected by differing cultural and social factors, which are discussed below. However, it is first worthwhile noting how the biomedical model defines differences between illness, disease, sickness and problems of living or 'predicaments' (Fig. 5.1).

The traditional medical model held that when people experienced symptoms – that is they felt ill – they sought medical help to identify a disease process. However, work done in the 1950s illustrated that many individuals with symptoms – even potentially serious ones – did not seek medical help. This was referred to as the 'clinical iceberg' to indicate that the majority of community illness was not seen by medical professionals. In addition, and somewhat conversely, it was noted that many people who do consult their general practitioner do so with trivial or minor complaints.

Ratio of symptom episodes to consultations
- Headache 184:1.
- Backache 52:1.
- Emotional problem 46:1.
- Abdominal pain 28:1.
- Sore throat 18:1.
- Chest pain 14:1.

Source: adapted from Banks et al. 1975 (as reproduced in Armstrong 1989)

Definition of illness, disease, sickness and predicaments (adapted from Hannay 1988)	Definition	Criterion
Illness	'the subjective component of disease as characterized by symptoms'	Subjective, medically and socially defined by doctor and patient
Disease	'an objective component confirmed by signs and investigations'	Objective, and medically defined
Sickness	'the behavioural part of illness – for example obtaining sick notes from the doctor, or adhering to the sick role'	Objective or subjective – defined both medically and socially
Predicaments	'problems of living or situations which are socially defined, but are not accepted by the medical community as being part of disease'	Objective or subjective, socially defined

Fig. 5.1 The definition of illness, disease, sickness and predicaments.

Illness behaviour

The notion of 'illness behaviour' was introduced in 1960 by Mechanic and Volkart to describe the ways in which symptoms were evaluated and acted upon or not acted upon by different kinds of individual. Mechanic (1978) outlined a number of variables that influence illness behaviour. Each variable may be considered in relation to its impact on others, and in its impact on the 'patient':

1. *Visibility, recognizability, or perceptual salience of signs and symptoms* – that is how obvious the symptoms are. Individuals with a sudden headache or acute abdominal pain may consult their GP more frequently than those with a slow-growing lump. In the same way, if illness causes a change in behaviour which is obvious to those close to the patient (e.g. expressed hallucinations), medical help may be sought more quickly than with an insidious change (e.g. increasing depression).

2. *The extent to which the symptoms are perceived as serious* – if a symptom is familiar, an individual may be more reluctant to visit a GP. Smokers may not attend a GP for a cough if they think 'it's just a smoker's cough', whereas a non-smoker might. Another example is if someone has a backache, and knows it was caused by heavy lifting, they may be less likely to attend the GP than if it had arisen 'out of the blue'.

3. *The extent to which symptoms disrupt family, work, and other social activities* – the heavy drinker with a family is more likely to present to health services due to pressure from those around him, than a solitary drinker. Similarly, if an individual is unable to play his weekly round of golf because of breathlessness, he may consult a GP before a less active individual in a similar stage of disease.

4. *The frequency of signs or symptoms, their persistence, or their frequency of recurrence* – frequent or persisting symptoms are more likely to lead to a consultation than rarely occurring ones.

5. *The tolerance threshold to the deviant signs and symptoms* – an individual's tolerance of pain and attitude towards it may determine when he consults a GP. This may be dependent on his cultural background. Zborowski (1952) showed that individuals of Irish or old-American descent were more stoical in their illness behaviour, in comparison to Italian and Jewish individuals who more readily courted sympathy. However, more recent studies do not support this work.

6. *Available information, knowledge and cultural assumptions and understandings of the individual* – lay individuals have a wide range of knowledge about medical conditions. Those who are unaware of how changes in their body may relate to disease processes may take longer to present to their GP. Those who are more fearful of diseases such as cancer, arthritis and birth defects tend to know more about them and may present earlier. For example, people who present to hospital within four hours of chest pain are more likely to see themselves as at risk from a heart attack, know more symptoms of a heart attack and are less likely to use drugs to treat their symptoms than those who delayed presentation. Psychosis in the lower social classes shows a greater tendency to present to health-care professionals via the courts or the police. Psychosis in the higher social classes tends to present via family, friends and self-referral.

7. *Basic needs that lead to denial* – anxiety, guilt and fear may lead individuals and their families to deny the existence of signs and symptoms of disease. However, this can be quite complex. Mechanic notes that whilst anxiety about cancer can lead to shorter delay in presentation, high levels of fear may lead to the opposite.

8. *Needs competing with illness responses* – individuals may feel that their symptoms do not warrant overriding other needs that may be more pressing.

9. *Competing possible interpretations that can be assigned to the symptoms once they are recognized* – friends and relatives may 'normalize' the symptoms of disease. Individuals who work long hours may not see tiredness as a symptom of illness – rather they expect it.

10. *Availability of treatment resources, physical proximity, and psychological and monetary costs of taking action* – the resumption of good health is not always a *supreme* priority – rather its attainment must be weighed against the other costs of going to see a doctor. The costs include:
    a. physical distance, time, money and effort
    b. stigma, social distance and feelings of humiliation
    c. self-blame and fear of being chastised for risky behaviour – for example, smoking

d. concern that the doctor will form a negative judgement about them if they present with something 'trivial'.

Source: adapted from Mechanic D 1978 Medical Sociology. New York: The Free Press, pp. 268–87.

The benefits of going to see the doctor are twofold:
1. Therapeutic benefit.
2. An endorsement of the 'sick role'.

Illness behaviour relates to the process by which individuals with symptoms seek (or don't seek) medical advice.

Zola (1973) identified five 'triggers' that may precipitate an individual with symptoms to consult a medical practitioner when they may not have otherwise:
1. The occurrence of an interpersonal crisis (e.g. a bereavement).
2. Perceived interference with social or personal relations.
3. 'Sanctioning' or pressure from others.
4. Perceived interference with vocational or physical activity.
5. 'Temporalizing of symptomatology' – the setting of deadlines before visiting the doctor, like 'if this headache comes back…' or 'if I still feel ill on Monday…'.

Lay referral and self-help

When an individual becomes aware of symptoms, they are presented with a number of options. They can:
1. Ignore them.
2. Self-medicate without consulting anyone else.
3. Consult non-medical individuals.
4. Consult a medical professional.

This section deals with options 2 and 3. Given the quantity of symptoms in the community that do not lead to a consultation, it seems apparent that individuals undertake a great deal of self-care. Most people have ways of dealing with bruises, muscular aches and pains, headaches, cuts and colds without needing to consult a doctor. Hannay has shown that the proportion of people with significant medical symptoms who do not consult a doctor is higher than the proportion of people with medical symptoms who do consult a doctor. It has been reported that twice as many people take non-prescription medicine as prescription medicine, and this self-medication was associated with a lower consultation rate. Encouraging self-care for self-limiting illnesses has clear benefits for health-care costs. However, Armstrong (1989) identified two problems that could arise if this policy were to be pursued too vigorously:

1. If people are encouraged to take responsibility for their health, they may also be seen as responsible for their illness. This 'victim-blaming' may be a particular problem for the lower socio-economic groups, as they are least likely to be able to 'look after' their health (see Ch. 7).
2. Health is not just an individual problem – rather it is contingent on social and economic factors as well. The placing of responsibility upon the individual may deflect attention from the responsibility of wider society to prevent social deprivation and inequality.

Up to three-quarters of patients consulting a medical practitioner will have already discussed their symptoms with some other person. This 'lay referral' system can either increase or decrease the likelihood of an individual seeking professional help.

One Scottish study showed high interlocking kinship and friendship networks 'inhibited' women from social class V seeking antenatal care.

Lay members may also take it upon themselves to initiate medical consultation. This is more likely if the symptoms are serious, or if the sufferer is incapable of self-help (e.g. a parent acting on behalf of a child, or a wife acting on behalf of a husband with epilepsy).

Beyond the 'lay referral' system exists a vast number of *self-help groups*. Self-help groups 'gather together people with a similar problem in order to help them by a personal approach, preferably to solve the problem, and where that is impossible, to teach them how to live with their constraints' (Damen et al. 2000).

The first such group, Alcoholics Anonymous, started in 1935. Today, groups exist for a vast range of illnesses including multiple sclerosis, hypertension, all manner of cancers and depression. By the end of the 70s there were thought to be over half a million self-help groups in the USA alone. Previously, many self-help groups were both characterized as and perceived themselves to be anti-medical – an alternative to professional medicine. This perception has broadly changed, and self-help groups are widely seen to be supplementary to professional assistance – able to act as expert bodies in the *experience* of diseases that is unrivalled by health-care professionals.

Self-help groups fulfil two main functions (Damen et al. 2000):

1. An informative aspect – they provide information about the condition, be this in leaflets, lectures, or through discussions with other individuals with the same condition.
2. An emotional aspect – they provide mechanisms to help the members to put their condition into perspective. Part of the role of such groups is to alleviate perceived stigma and aid narrative reconstruction (p. 98).

In general, self-help groups are seen as beneficial – reducing stress, increasing patient control and improving self-esteem. In particular:

- Self-help groups are, next to family, the most important pillars for the chronically ill.
- The long-term impact of group membership, for example in cancer patients, can lead to a significant reduction in anxiety and depression.

However, there have been some studies that have found the supportive or emotional side to self-help groups to be lacking.

- One study, reporting on newly diagnosed cancer patients, found that, although 66% used other patients as a source of support, only 39% found this to be a positive source.
- A number of factors could lead to negative experiences in such groups:
  - the presence of disruptive individual members at meetings
  - the experience of loss when members left
  - the potential for member dependency
  - individuals feeling threatened by the open communication.
- Self-help groups for breast cancer have been found to be beneficial in relation to the informative aspect; however, in practical aspects of how to cope with breast cancer, many people found the emotional support aspect was less useful, for the following reasons (Damen et al. 2000):

  - they perceived that such support from strangers was for people who had few other social ties (such as no partner or family)
  - they felt no need for such support
  - they wished to 'leave their cancer behind them'
  - they felt there existed too great a gap of severity between themselves and the other group members
  - they felt there existed too great a gap of age between themselves and the other group members.

Aside from self-help, individuals may choose to visit practitioners of alternative medicine or use complementary medicine.

Alternative and complementary medicine

As the names suggest, alternative is used as a replacement for conventional medicine and complementary is used alongside conventional medicine, often through referral (see http://nccam.nci.nih.gov/health/whatiscam for a full definition). It has been estimated that alternative medicine is growing five times as fast as orthodox or conventional medicine. Alternative medicine can be seen as part of a wider societal shift of attitude towards natural and 'organic' choices: this includes the green movements and the increased interest in organic foods versus pesticide-treated foods, holistic versus mechanistic approaches and so on. Such popular support for alternative and complementary medicine has led to political support – with the appointment of junior ministers with responsibility for alternative medicine and the unveiling of plans to set up the Complementary Medical Council along the same lines as the General Medical Council.

There has also been a shift in perception by the medical community itself – with complementary medicine increasingly being practised in conventional medical settings – particularly with regards to acupuncture for pain, and massage, music therapy and relaxation therapy for mild anxiety and depression. This has largely been ascribed to the increasing amount of evidence in favour of certain complementary therapies.

Proponents of alternative and complementary medicine argue that the following benefits are offered:

- Care is health and not disease oriented.
- It respects the autonomy of the patient.
- It allows freedom of choice.
- It promotes self-treatment.

- It encourages the patient to take on some individual responsibility for the outcome of the procedure and healing.

For patients, the common reasons given for attending a practitioner of alternative or complementary medicine include:

- A greater amount of time and continuity in the consultation: this allows the development of a deeper therapeutic relationship than the kind that can be forged in the average GP or hospital consultation.
- The attention to personality and personal experience: treatment is 'individualized' in the sense of making it dependent on the patient's emotions, psychology and response to illness – rather than focused on the disease itself.
- Greater patient involvement: the patient is able to choose the type of therapist that they think would suit them; for example, a homeopathist, reflexologist, acupuncture practitioner and so on. There is also the greater sense of being active in one's own treatment as compared to conventional medicine, which can make patients adopt a rather passive role to treatment.
- Hope: patients may come to alternative or complementary medicine after having tried all that conventional medicine has to offer.
- Touch: many of the alternative or complementary therapies involve a degree of physical contact with the patient that would perhaps be out of place in conventional medicine. This aspect can be important in facilitating a more open and trusting relationship between patient and practitioner.
- Dealing with ill-defined symptoms: alternative or complementary medicine may be better placed to deal with non-specific syndromes and symptoms; for example, chronic fatigue and irritable bowel syndrome.
- Making sense of illness: alternative or complementary medicine may provide explanations for patients' conditions that they find easy to understand. The treatment may fit with a patient's own personal beliefs or seem less threatening than 'orthodox' medicine by presenting a 'natural' alternative. The objectivity of such explanations may on occasion be questionable; however, if they accord with the prior beliefs of the patients, they may be beneficial.

- Spiritual and existential concerns: such concerns are often not addressed by conventional practitioners. However, one study has shown that 66% of Americans would like their doctors to be aware of their religious or spiritual beliefs. Practitioners of alternative or complementary medicine may be more comfortable addressing these sorts of issues.

The above reasons represent a number of 'pull' factors towards alternative and complementary medicine; however, patients may experience a number of 'push' or negative factors that lead to a loss of faith in conventional medicine. These include being less confident about the conventional medicine, and less satisfied by it, as well as being more sceptical of its efficacy.

The negative aspects of alternative and complementary medicine include:

- Safety and competence – a lack of regulation may lead to unqualified practitioners. In addition, herbal medications are not subject to the same level of testing as conventional drugs – even though they may contain pharmacologically active components with significant side effects.
- Guilt and blame – when patients are encouraged to feel more responsible for their own health they may be made to feel guilty for their past activities that have led to ill health, or to feel blame for not getting better.
- Financial risk – there is a danger of exploiting the vulnerable who are willing to try multiple alternative or complementary therapies to find a successful outcome.
- Missed diagnosis or delayed presentation – conventional practitioners worry that alternative practitioners may miss serious diagnoses. This is only a risk in alternative medicine where it replaces the conventional medicine; however, most patients are most likely to consult conventional prior to alternative or complementary therapy.
- Conflicting advice – may lead to the abandonment of conventional therapy with potentially serious consequences.
- Interference with conventional medicines.

Normality, the sick role, deviance and stigma in disease

When individuals talk about health, there are perhaps three commonly understood components of what health is. These are (Blaxter 1990):

1. A positive element: fitness and well-being.
2. A functional element: an ability to cope with day to day life.
3. A negative element: an absence of illness.

All these elements are overtly dependent on *social* values and criteria. However, when individuals talk about disease, it is in terms of *biological* criteria. Why does such a difference exist? A definition of 'disease' as a group noun is more difficult than defining the criteria of individual diseases. This may be because:

- There is no agreed definition of disease.
- Some diseases do not appear to have an apparent biological basis; for example, some psychiatric diseases.
- If disease is simply some pathological state – that is some biological set of conditions – how can it be distinguished from a non-diseased biological state? That is, what differentiates a 'normal' biological state from an abnormal one?

Normality in medicine may be decided on a number of bases as outlined below.

Statistical basis One example of this is the 'normal' range of blood biochemistry, which is based on samples of the 'healthy' population and will fall in a 'normal' or Gaussian distribution. Levels that are outside a certain number of standard deviations from the mean are considered to be abnormal – even if they are not associated with symptoms. There are a number of problems with this approach:

1. The cut-off point may be somewhat arbitrary; for example, diagnosis of diabetes or hypertension relies on what is effectively an arbitrary point in a spectrum of disease.
2. Certain biological states might be considered to be disease states, yet are statistically 'normal'; for example, the presence of atheroma is 'normal' in Western populations, but is still considered to be a disease process.
3. Certain biological states might *not* be considered to be a disease state, yet be statistically 'abnormal'; for example, being 7 ft tall, or having a 'genius' IQ.

Bio-statistical basis This is a variation of the statistical basis that aims to find a way around the problems mentioned above. This theory still holds that disease is an objective status, that not only can it be defined regardless of whether the patient 'feels' ill, but regardless of whether or not society negatively or positively values that particular biological state. This theory has been advocated by Boorse (1975).

He asserts that disease is not an evaluative concept; rather, disease is an abnormality that hinders the attainment of 'natural goals'. An analysis of a large enough sample will lead to a bio-statistical analysis of what constitutes a natural and thus factual goal. This goal becomes the basis for judgements on what is and what is not a disease. He claims that:

> An organism is healthy at any moment in proportion as it is not diseased; and a disease is a type of internal state of the organism which:
> 1. Interferes with the performance of some natural function, i.e. some species-typical contribution to survival and reproduction, characteristic of the organism's age; and
> 2. Is not simply in the nature of the species, i.e. is either atypical of the species or, if typical, mainly due to environmental causes.
>
> (Boorse 1976)

However, a fundamental problem still exists. Namely, Boorse wishes to use terms like 'natural function' and 'biological disadvantage' as objective, descriptive terms, which are then used to elicit what doctors *ought* to treat without a need for moral analysis. However, it seems that inherent within the terms there is a moral judgement. 'Natural function' is that which is 'good' and 'biological disadvantage' is 'bad'. This assumption is not obviously true. As Toon (1981) writes: 'This tendency to find moral values creeping in under the cloak of a scientific definition is a central problem in the definition of disease, and it merely leads to confusion.' It is thus more prudent to accept that 'disease' in both its professional and its colloquial usage incorporates a degree of moral evaluation.

Normative basis This view holds that normality is defined in the way in which society finds acceptable or desirable. It is often equivalent with those that are statistically normal, but not always. Some of the advantages of this approach are:

- It better accords with many of our intuitions about disease.
- By defining normality in relation to socially accepted or desired criteria, disease becomes those states with socially deleterious consequences.
- Psychiatric disease, such as 'mania', is more readily understandable as a state that by (our) collective values is considered undesirable – even if the patient doesn't consider himself to be ill. Another example is homosexuality which, until the 1980s, was generally considered a mental illness.

Conditions such as 'dyslexia' only exist as 'diseases' in literate societies – the same biological state may exist in pre-literate cultures, but it isn't a disease because it doesn't confer any social disadvantage.

The sick role

With this conception of disease as a socially definable phenomenon, the sick role and illness can be understood as forms of social deviancy (deviancy in the sense of being different from what is the social 'norm', rather than in a pejorative sense or in the sense that the 'deviant' is morally responsible for 'not being normal'). As can certain diseases that carry with them considerable stigma – which essentially is social disapproval.

Prior to the 1950s, deviance was simply used to describe those who were responsible for behaving in a way that did not accord with social and cultural norms, for example youth crime. Parsons (1951) defined deviance on the grounds that 'it disrupts the social system by inhibiting people's performance of their customary or normal social roles'. The sick role, according to Parsons, has the function of minimizing such social disruption, controlling the deviant illness behaviour. The sick role consists of two rights and two responsibilities (or duties).

The rights are:
1. The sick are not obliged to perform their normal social roles.
2. The sick are not considered responsible for their own state.

The responsibilities are:
1. The sick are obliged to want to get well as soon as possible.
2. To consult and cooperate with medical experts.

Failure to successfully carry out the responsibilities of the sick role means that the sick may forfeit the rights associated with their role. Someone who appears not to want to get well may be considered a malingerer or a hypochondriac. Someone who doesn't cooperate with medical experts is seen as non-compliant. The non-compliant patient may be seen as responsible for his illness in a way that other patients are not; for example, the patient who continues to smoke after bypass surgery.

The sick role is in general a temporary role into which all people can be admitted. The gatekeepers to the sick role are doctors who decide whether or not individuals have a disease. In doing so they must draw upon general and objective criteria. However, it is possible to have a medical diagnosis, but not be admitted into the 'sick role'. For example, many people in Africa may suffer from constant diagnosable medical conditions such as malaria or malnutrition. However, because their economies cannot support non-productive individuals for any length of time, they are not considered sick and must carry out their social roles.

The main functions of the sick role are:
1. To control illness.
2. To reduce the disruptive effects on the social systems by returning the ill to good health as quickly as possible.

Labelling

Labelling refers to the process whereby individual characteristics are identified by others and given a negative label.

The act of making a diagnosis is the process by which people become 'patients' and are labelled as ill or deviant. In this sense, labelling *creates* disease. This shouldn't be confused with *causing* disease, which it doesn't. Rather it enables the normal to be reaffirmed and the deviant to be identified. Labelling serves to delineate the boundaries of what are considered to be normal social values and behaviour.

Secondary deviance refers to the changes in behaviour as a result of labelling an illness (primary deviance). Strong social attitudes or stereotypes about how a blind, epileptic or alcoholic person should act may lead to self-fulfilling prophecies. The pressure upon patients derives from the expectations associated with the label (or diagnosis) a patient has been given. The blind may be seen as quiet and docile, the alcoholic as unkempt and incorrigible. People they encounter, and even medical professionals who deal with them, may present such stereotypic attitudes to the individual patients. This reactive attitude towards them may lead the patients to conform to the stereotype imposed upon them (either by others or self-imposed because they believe such stereotypical behaviour is appropriate for their illness).

The idea of secondary deviance has been most controversial in the field of psychiatry. Three main views exist as to the impact of labelling primary deviance, and secondary deviance:
1. *Psychiatric disease is a consequence of the labelling of primary deviance* – this view claimed that psychiatric illness only existed because certain behaviours were labelled as 'illness'; 'real' psychiatric illness did not exist.

2. *Psychiatric illness is a consequence of the labelling of primary deviance and the resulting secondary deviance* – this view holds that psychiatrists identify a slightly unusual behaviour in individuals (which is still within the normal range) and label it as psychiatric disease (that is primary deviance). The result of the labelling (that is secondary deviance) is the induction of the mental illness that was first diagnosed.

3. *Psychiatric illness can be exacerbated by labelling and secondary deviance* – this view holds that labelling and secondary deviance lead to some behaviours that are 'abnormal'. This is most evident in patients who have lived in institutions for many years. Such patients may develop certain behaviours that, whilst they are normal behaviours within the institute, may be seen as incongruous in the 'normal' world.

Stigma

The concept of *stigma* requires us to accept that the labels given in a medical diagnosis have a significance beyond the medical consultation and into wider society. 'Stigmatizing conditions [are] those that set their possessors apart from "normal" people [and] mark them as socially unacceptable or inferior beings' (Scambler 2003). Some of the most stigmatizing

The process of labelling and stigma involves a *negative* evaluation about a condition or its causes with respect to what is considered to be socially normal and acceptable.

conditions are those that are generally visible; for example being deaf, or blind, or being seen to have an epileptic fit, or being an amputee. However, many other non-visible conditions also have considerable stigma attached to them by virtue of strong social emotions related to the condition; for example, cancer (and the associated fear of dying), colostomies (and the social taboo about handling faeces) and HIV/AIDS (and the 'moral' condemnation of homosexuality and/or intravenous drug use) (Fig. 5.2).

Goffman (1963) described several strategies that a person with a stigmatizing condition could pursue. He described stigmatizing conditions as either:

- *Discrediting* – if they were obviously visible (for example being in a wheelchair).

The four phases of the HIV stigma trajectory	
At risk: pre-stigma and the 'worried well'	This does not correspond to a stage of the disease trajectory. It denotes a time of uncertainty when an individual thinks behaviours might have put him at risk of HIV. He may cope through denial or disassociation. Much depends on the support available. The phase may end with testing for HIV.
Diagnosis: confronting an altered identity	An individual may be diagnosed early or late in the disease trajectory. A typical stress response involves disbelief, numbness and denial, followed by anger, acute turmoil, disruptive anxiety and depressive symptoms. Identity and self-esteem may be threatened, stigma becomes salient, and decisions on disclosure have to be negotiated.
Latent: living between health and illness	This is when the disease is asymptomatic and perhaps at its least disruptive. Individuals may normalize, conceal and even deny their positivity. They may choose to pass as normal, thereby avoiding enacted stigma, but felt stigma can exact a heavy price.
Manifest: passage to social and physical death	There may be no fixed disease course because of widespread individual variation. However, there are fewer symptom-free periods and opportunistic infections accumulate. Stigma tends to be less salient as matters surrounding social and biological death become paramount. Intense felt stigma may, nevertheless, be associated with isolation and withdrawal as means of concealing 'abominations of the body'. Courtesy stigma may extend to carers who hesitate to reveal cause of death.

Source: Alonzo A, Reynolds N 1995 Stigma, HIV and AIDS: an exploration and elaboration of a stigma strategy. Social Sciences in Medicine 41: 303–15

Fig. 5.2 The four phases of the HIV stigma trajectory.

or

- *Discreditable* – if they were relatively hidden (for example HIV).

Having a stigmatizing condition that was discrediting limited one's options; however, the patient with the discreditable condition had the option of trying to keep the condition hidden. Coping with stigmatizing conditions could be achieved in one of the following ways:

1. Passing – by trying to 'pass as normal'. This would depend on the degree and nature of the stigmatizing condition. Problems that might occur revolve around the need for various forms of deception and the risk of being exposed.
2. Covering – a person with a discrediting condition could still try to hide the condition from view, or avoid situations where it is particularly obvious.
3. Withdrawal – at extremes, individuals may withdraw from social circumstances where attention may be drawn to their stigmatizing condition.

Scambler and Hopkins (1986) identified a distinction between two components of stigma:

1. Felt stigma – the shame associated with the condition, and the fear of being discriminated against because of the imputed cultural unacceptability or inferiority.
2. Enacted stigma – actual discrimination of this nature.

The same authors noted that often the felt stigma is greater than the actual or enacted stigma, and led to greater disruption of people's lives (in attempting to hide their medical condition) than probably would have been the case of enduring the enacted stigma.

The doctor–patient relationship

Morgan (2003) refers to the meeting of patients with their doctors as the 'essential unit of medical practice'. There are estimated to be over half a million consultations between patients and GPs in the UK every day. The utility and success of these consultations depends on the competence and expertise of the doctor, and the social relationship between doctor and patient.

How the doctor–patient relationship is changing

In the 18th century, physicians treated aristocrats. The status difference and the need for physicians to

The doctor–patient relationship
- The doctor–patient relationship reflects and reinforces wider social relations and structural inequalities – especially those of gender, 'race' and socio-economic class.
- The relationship and values maintained within them form a key dimension to social control.
- Traditionally, the view of the patient has been neglected.
- The quality of the doctor–patient relationship impacts on the health outcomes.

compete amongst themselves meant that the doctor–patient relationship was characterized by doctors attempting to please their patients. The lack of technical knowledge meant the doctor's role was that of attending to symptoms and experiences.

Throughout the 19th century, doctors found themselves more commonly practising charitable medicine in the newly created public or voluntary hospitals. The biomedical model of illness was emerging allowing doctors to treat the pathological lesion within their patients who were often their social inferiors and more passive. It became normal for the doctor to occupy the dominant role within the doctor–patient consultation.

The 1950s were characterized by the paternalistic doctor-centred approach typified by the Parsons model (see p. 90).

From the 1960s onwards there has been a general trend toward a relationship involving greater patient participation. In sociological terms this has been described by relationships of *mutuality* rather than paternalism. In ethical terms this has been discussed in terms of patient *autonomy*.

In 1992 (updated in 1995) the Patient's Charter was introduced. This has formally given patients a number of rights and also affirmed what standards the public can expect from the NHS. The rights patients are entitled to include:

- A clear explanation of treatment, its alternatives and associated risks.
- A full investigation of any complaints.
- Waiting lists of a maximum of 18 months.

Patients can also expect the following standards:
- To be seen within 30 minutes of an appointment time.
- To be seen immediately at A&E or have need for treatment assessed.
- To have their privacy, dignity, religious and cultural beliefs respected.

All the current changes seem to be increasing the *consumer* power of the patient. This is partly reflected by the increase in litigation.

At the moment, the patient-centred or relationship-centred approach is being advocated (see p. 92). However, the paternalistic model is still prevalent.

Models of the doctor–patient relationship

As mentioned in the previous section, Parsons (1951) was one of the first to deal with the relationship between doctors and patients. Parsons believed that social functioning was achieved in part by the fulfilment of social roles – each of which had certain prescribed or expected behaviours. This meant that we know what to expect when interacting with mothers, teachers and doctors, and how we in turn are expected to behave in the role of children, pupils and patients. Just as Parsons held that the sick role had certain rights and responsibilities, he believed the doctor role had a number of rights and obligations as well. These are summarized in Figure 5.3.

Parsons viewed the sick role as:
- *Temporary* – only for as long as it takes to get better.
- *Universal* – the obligations and rights apply to all regardless of gender, race, or socio-economic class.

Parsons thought of the doctor's role as complementary – but not equal – to the sick role. The asymmetry in the relationship was not thought to be problematic due to the expectations or obliged attitudes of the doctor, namely:
- *Affective neutrality* – to remain emotionally detached and objective in the diagnosis and treatment of disease.
- *Universalism* – to treat patients equally.
- *Functional specificity* – the doctor should be concerned only with those matters that are of direct medical relevance to the patient.

This is of course an 'ideal' model of the doctor–patient relationship. Everyday reality will depart from this ideal.

Armstrong (1989) outlines three different types of doctor–patient relationship models:

Fig. 5.3 The role of doctor and patient.

The role of doctor and patient	
Patient: sick role	**Doctor: professional role**
Rights	**Expectations**
1. Allowed to shed normal social role	1. Apply a high degree of skill and knowledge to the problem of illness
2. Regarded as not being responsible for illness	2. Act for the welfare of patient and community
Obligations	3. Be objective and emotionally detached
1. Must want to get well	4. Be guided by professional practice
2. Should seek medical help and cooperate with doctor	**Rights**
	1. Granted right to examine patients and enquire into intimate areas of physical and personal life
	2. Granted considerable autonomy in professional practice
	3. Occupies position of authority in relation to patient

Source: Adapted from Parsons T 1951 The Social System. Glencoe, IL: Free Press, as reproduced by Morgan M The doctor–patient relationship. In: Scambler G (ed.) 2003 Sociology as Applied to Medicine, 5th edn. Edinburgh: Saunders, p. 51

A comparison of Parsons'
doctor–patient relationship and
the GMC's Duties of a Doctor.

Parsons (1951)
- Apply a high level of knowledge.
- Be guided by professional practice.
- Act for the welfare of patient and community rather than self-interest.
- Be objective and emotionally detached (not judge patient's behaviour in terms of personal value system or become emotionally involved with them).

GMC (2001)
- Keep your professional knowledge and skills up to date.
- Make the care of your patient your first concern.
- Make sure that your personal beliefs do not prejudice your patients' care.

1. Consensual models – such as the Parsons model – where both the doctor and the patient have the same goals framed within the perspective of the biomedical model. That is, even if the doctor and patient don't agree on how best to produce a cure, they have agreed on their aims – specifically to produce a cure.

2. Conflict models – where the patient and the doctor have different agendas and perspectives that may often be in conflict – and are often not addressed.

3. Negotiation models – where it is recognized within the consultation that the doctor has a biomedical agenda and the patient a psychosocial agenda, and attempts are made to understand the patient's view and integrate their lay beliefs into a workable plan for treatment.

These models represent different types of relationship between doctor and patient. The Parsons model is a *paternalistic* one; ultimately, the patient in the 'sick role' is obliged to cooperate with the doctor. Other types of relationship occur when different levels of power and control are exercised by doctors and patients (Fig. 5.4).

In the *paternalistic* relationship the doctor is authoritative, acting in much the same way as a parent deciding what is best for their child. The agenda for the consultation is determined by the doctor, who assumes patient values without enquiring after them. For example, a doctor may assume all patients who have a sore throat desire antibiotics, when in fact they may simply want reassurance, or vice versa. Recognition of patient autonomy means that consultations are leaning away from this paternalistic approach, although it may still be the most prevalent style of consultation. However, some sections of the population may prefer the paternalistic approach, such as the elderly.

Fig. 5.4 Types of doctor–patient relationships.

Types of doctor–patient relationships

Patient control	Physician control	
	LOW	HIGH
LOW	Default	Paternalism
Goals and agenda	Unclear	Physician set
Patient values	Unclear	Assumed
Physician's role	Unclear	Guardian
HIGH	Consumerist	Mutuality
Goals and agenda	Patient set	Negotiated
Patient values	Unexamined	Jointly examined
Physician's role	Technical consultant	Advisor

Source: adapted from Roter D 2000 The enduring and evolving nature of the patient–physician relationship. Patient Education and Counseling 39(5–15): 6

Paternalism may also be more prevalent in other cultures (for example Japan is reported to have a more paternalistic medical profession).

A relationship of *mutuality* sees doctors and patients in a 'meeting of experts', the doctor with clinical skills and knowledge, and the patient with experience and expectations of the illness and possibly complex ideas about its causation. This is the sort of relationship that is encouraged in the Western practice of modern medicine.

A *consumerist* relationship may develop if the patient becomes demanding, and the doctor acquiesces to their demands, for example for antibiotics for a viral infection or an unnecessary referral. This type of relationship is more prevalent where patients are paying to see the doctor. This type of consultation is characterized by the patient setting the agenda, and the doctor acting as little more than a facilitator. The patient's values are unexamined by the physician, which may lead to the patient having an ongoing false impression of her condition.

A *default* relationship occurs when neither the doctor nor the patient takes an active role in the consultation. The danger here is that the consultation is undirected and the appropriate decisions may not be made.

Of course, these types of consultation represent extremes; a single consultation may contain a mixture of styles, the doctor being paternalistic with an issue she considers important, and the patient being more demanding with others.

The patient-centred consultation

A 'patient-centred' consultation style is increasingly advocated in all settings, but especially in primary care where there is a high degree of psychological and social aspects to the consultation. What then is 'patient-centredness'?

Mead and Bower (2002) describe the following five dimensions of 'patient-centred care':

1. The biopsychosocial perspective – this takes into account the biomedical, psychological and social factors that lead to a patient consulting.
2. The 'patient-as-person' – this dimension invites the doctor to consider the personal meaning of the illness for that individual patient.
3. Sharing power and responsibility – the aim of this perspective is to remind doctors to be sensitive to patient preferences, and understand the reasons and values that guide their actions.

4. The therapeutic alliance – this aims to develop common goals and agendas that take into account both the patient's and the doctor's preferences. The idea of developing a mutual goal is that it is more likely to be achieved than one that is simply dictated by the doctor.
5. The 'doctor-as-person' – this aspect reflects a need for doctors to be introspective to a degree – being aware of how their own personal qualities and their subjectivity affect their practice of medicine. Doctors' assumptions of patients' preferences may have more influence than the actual preferences of patients – resulting in actions deemed unnecessary by the doctor and unwanted by the patient.

The term 'patient-centred consultation' is used to draw attention to the importance of the patient in the consultation. However, it is characterized by *mutuality* as described above – where both patient and doctor are partners in the process treating the patient – rather than a consumerist relationship, which the term 'patient-centred consultation' might suggest. Some authors prefer to describe this as '*relationship-centred care*' in order to avoid this problem and to recognize the importance of the reciprocal relationship between the doctor and the patient, and the integration of the biomedical and real-life or personal perspective of the patient. Such consultations (whatever we choose to call them) are characterized by being:

- Medically functional – the consultation must work within the framework of a health-care system. History-taking, examination, diagnosis and treatment are expected of the consultation.
- Informative for the patient – in general, patients want to know as much information as possible about their conditions. Some studies have shown that when patients are better informed (for example what the symptoms of a heart attack are) they are more likely to seek appropriate medical care.
- Facilitative – that is the doctor should aim to elicit the full concerns of the patient and their pre-consultation agenda. The majority of patients do not discuss their full agenda during a single consultation, the consequences of which can be a number of misunderstandings.
- Responsive – in addition to being experts in health, doctors need to respond to patients at a human level – offering 'support, empathy, concern and legitimation' (Roter 2000) to patients. This helps to

build a rapport with the patient, and make them feel that they are being listened to and understood.

- Participatory – this implies that patients should take a responsible and active role in medical decision-making. The degree to which they are able to do this will be dependent on the patient's desire to be involved in their health care and the encouragement they receive from their doctor to do so.

Patients' agendas

The patients' agendas are their ideas, concerns and expectations. Agendas may include:

- Symptoms – patient may have multiple symptoms, but through embarrassment or uncertainty about the significance of symptoms, may not mention all of them.
- A request for a prescription/or a desire not to have a prescription – some patients may feel that a prescription represents a positive step towards treating illness, others may feel a prescription treats the symptoms without addressing the cause of illness.
- Previous self-treatment.
- A request for diagnosis.
- Theories about diagnosis.
- Reporting of side effects.
- Worries about diagnosis or prognosis – patients often have questions about their health, or need clarifications, but feel unable to ask.
- Social concerns.

Conflict in the doctor–patient relationship

As mentioned above, conflict may arise in a consultation due to different expectations – the doctor wishing to pursue biomedical goals, and the patient seeking the resolution of a social problem and a degree of reassurance. However, conflict may also be imposed on the relationship by a number of other factors:

- Competing demands of many patients for limited resources such as doctors' time.
- The problem of uncertainty about diagnosis and treatment.

- The knowledge that some diagnoses are unhelpful, and some treatments ineffective.
- The conflict between the present and future interests of the patient; for example, should the doctor reveal a poor prognosis now?
- The conflict between the patient's interests and those of his/her family or the state; for example, whether to inform the DVLA about a newly diagnosed epileptic.
- The inability to resolve social problems, such as damp housing, or problem neighbours, which lead to stress and the somatic symptoms.
- The conflict with the doctor's other roles; for example, the doctor's role as a mother and her responsibility to collect her children from nursery.

Resolving conflict in the doctor–patient relationship

- *Doctor's practice style*: The doctor's practice style can be described as doctor-centred or patient-centred. The doctor-centred style is paternalistic and is characterized by the use of closed questions, and active information gathering (for example 'do you have any pain?' and 'is the pain burning or stabbing?'). The patient may be interrupted and is expected to be passive. The consultation is limited to the medical problem the patient has and may not address any psychosocial concerns of the patient. By contrast, the patient-centred approach is characterized by open-ended questions (for example 'how do you feel?' and 'tell me about the pain'). The process requires greater patient participation and reflects a relationship of *mutuality* (see p. 92).
- *Influence of time*: Lack of time is often cited by doctors as hindering their attendance to the psychosocial concerns of patients, and 'feeling hurried' is a reason given by patients for not mentioning all their symptoms (or sometimes their major complaint). However, a doctor's practice style may have more important influence on the content of consultations. By adopting a patient-centred approach (which does tend to take longer) doctors are more likely to fully understand the patient's perspective and provide a treatment that is acceptable to both parties. The suggestion has been made that by initially spending extra time with the patient, the doctor may reduce subsequent visits and increase compliance, so saving time in the long run, and benefiting the patient's health. It has also been suggested that a doctor's practice style, rather than length of consultation, is a better predictor of patient satisfaction and the eliciting of complete patient agendas.

- *Influence of structural context*: Consultations with the same patient may vary between the primary and secondary care settings. Patients may adopt a more passive role when seeing a specialist or in an acute setting, but prefer a more active role when consulting the GP. Private patients may be more demanding in their consultations, and their doctors, who are more reliant on the goodwill of the patient, may be more passive.
- *Patients' expectations and participation*: the role the patient takes may change as the consultation process goes on. It has been reported that patients who were passive in their first consultation had increased participation and were more critical by the third.

- *Communications skills*: Communications skills are important in eliciting information from patients in order to get a good history, discovering the patient's concerns, and in conveying information back to the patient about the cause of their illness and its proposed management. The following considerations may be of use in improving these aspects and in avoiding any misunderstanding (see also Fig. 5.5):
  – Removing physical barriers (such as desks) between the doctor and patient
  – Use of body language (maintaining eye contact, adopting a relaxed, but not too relaxed posture, appropriate facial expressions)
  – Use of appropriate sounds, for example 'uh-huh'

Fig. 5.5 Categories of misunderstanding in relation to prescribing.

Categories of misunderstanding in relation to prescribing

Britten et al. (2000) studied the sorts of misunderstandings in prescribing that occurred in general practice. Of 35 consultations, 28 had some degree of misunderstanding. The common reasons are outlined below:

1. Patient information remains unknown to the doctor, for example:
   a. The patient doesn't mention previous medical history (e.g. side effects from a previously tried medication) wrongly believing the doctor is already aware of it
   b. The doctor has an inaccurate perception of what the patient wants (e.g. the doctor assumes the patient wants antibiotics, when in fact they merely want reassurance)
   c. The doctor is unaware that the patient is taking over-the-counter medication (either due to failure to ask, or active concealment)

2. Doctor information remains unknown to the patient, for example:
   a. Patient does not understand why they have been prescribed a certain medication and therefore takes it incorrectly or not at all
   b. Patient is unaware of the correct dose or is confused about the correct dose

3. Conflicting information given, for example:
   a. The patient is confused by receiving different information from the doctor and other sources; for example, the hospital specialist or the pharmacist

4. Failure of communication about the doctor's diagnosis:
   a. The patient may not understand, remember or accept a diagnosis (for example, a patient who was receiving two sorts of injections stops taking the wrong one, because he/she misunderstood which one the doctor had advised him/her to stop)
   b. The patient may not understand how treatment can be prescribed in the absence of a diagnosis

5. Relationship factors:
   a. The doctor may write a prescription, not because he thinks it is necessary, but in order to preserve a relationship (for example either because it is a repeat prescription by a partner in the practice the doctor does not wish to challenge, or in order to maintain a good relationship with the patient who desires a prescription)

The misunderstandings in prescribing tended to be associated with a patient's lack of participation in the consultation, and in many cases were based on inaccurate assumptions by both doctors and patients

Source: Britten N et al. 2000 Misunderstandings in prescribing decisions in general practice. British Medical Journal 320: 485 (Box 1)

– Using 'open-ended' questions
– Giving instructions and advice before other information – this is known as primary effect – people are more likely to remember the first bits of information they are given
– Use of simple, clear, specific instructions
– Repetition – this can be used to clarify parts of the history, or to ensure the patient is confident about how to take their medication
– Providing written information – booklets or leaflets that are relevant
– Asking if the patient has any questions

Compliance and concordance

Alongside the shift in attitudes about the doctor–patient relationship, from doctor-centred to patient-centred, there has been a shift in the attitude towards those patients with differing agendas to those of their doctors.

Compliance has been described as 'following doctor's orders' – and thus non-compliance has been used to describe any behaviour that is seen as disobedient, for example not taking prescribed medication. Other terms such as adherence and cooperation have been used, but were also criticized for not being far away enough in meaning from compliance.

Qualitative studies have shown that the three main reasons for non-compliance are:
• Lack of knowledge or understanding.
• Unpleasant side effects from medication.
• Perceived or real stigma: feeling that taking the medicine isn't 'normal', so patient keeps testing out whether they can stop taking drug and become 'normal'.

In 1997, a report published by the Royal Pharmaceutical Society of Great Britain's working party on medicine-taking recommended that 'concordance' should replace the term 'compliance'. Concordance is 'a process of prescribing and medicine-taking based on partnership' (Medicines partnership) between the doctor and the patient.

The need for this sort of approach has arisen subsequent to research showing that many people, especially those with chronic conditions, do not take their medicines as prescribed. Two-thirds of older patients prescribed statin for coronary artery disease will have given up treatment within two years, and half of people diagnosed with hypertension do not take the drugs that, as prescribed, may benefit their health. These patients are denied real health benefits and it is suggested that informed discussion within

the concordance model will go some way to remedying this problem.

Compliance and concordance
• Compliance refers to a specific patient behaviour – namely did the patient do what was requested by the doctor?
• Concordance refers to a consultation process between a health-care professional and a patient and is based on the ethos of a shared approach to decision-making rather than paternalism.

The advocates of concordance suggest that it is different from compliance, adherence and cooperation, in that it promotes a sharing of power in the doctor–patient relationship. Concordance recognizes the patient's expertise in their experience of illness and response to treatment. While this expertise is different from that of the clinician's, it is of equal relevance and value in terms of deciding on best management. The idea is that doctor and patient will embark on joint decision-making processes to reach a clinically effective treatment that is acceptable to the patient's beliefs, values and ideas about their disease. It is hoped that the ethos of concordance will lead to less drug wastage and fewer hospital admissions due to the iatrogenic effects of drugs.

Joint decision-making of this sort requires certain competencies of both doctors and patients (Fig. 5.6). Joint decision-making of this kind is considered to be important because it leads to (Cox 2003):
• Improved satisfaction with care.
• Increased knowledge of the condition and treatment.
• Increased adherence.
• Improved health outcomes.
• Fewer medication-related problems.

However, it has also been suggested that concordance may not be as successful as anticipated. It is reported that:
1. Up to 80% of information given to patients is forgotten at once.

Fig. 5.6 Competencies for doctors and patients to facilitate joint decision-making.

Competencies for doctors and patients to facilitate joint decision-making

Competencies for doctors	Competencies for patients
1. Develop a partnership with the patient	1. Define (for oneself) the preferred doctor–patient relationship
2. Establish the patient's preferences for information (amount and format)	2. Find a doctor and establish, develop, and adapt a partnership
3. Establish the patient's preference for the role in decision-making and any uncertainty	3. Articulate (for oneself) health problems, feelings, beliefs, and expectations in an objective and systematic manner
4. Ascertain and respond to patient's ideas, concerns and expectations	4. Communicate with the physician in order to understand and share relevant information clearly and at the appropriate time in the medical interview
5. Identify choices and evaluate the research evidence in relation to the individual patient	5. Access information
6. Present (or direct patient to) evidence, taking into account (2) and (3). Help patient to reflect on and assess the impact of alternative decisions with regard to his/her lifestyle and values	6. Evaluate information
7. Make or negotiate a decision in partnership with the patient and resolve any conflict	7. Negotiate decisions, give feedback, resolve conflict, agree on an action plan
8. Agree an action plan and complete arrangements for follow-up	

Source: Towle A & Godolphin W 1999 Framework for teaching and learning informed shared decision making. British Medical Journal 319:766–71

2. Half of the information that does remain is incorrect.
3. Leaflets and other aids may increase satisfaction and knowledge but rarely improve physical outcome.
4. Even if patients are well informed, decisions may be wholly irrational.

Other authors have commented that:
- Patients tended to overestimate the risks of common complications.
- Patients could not assess the meaning of outcome statistics.
- Some patients had little interest in choice while others were too emotionally compromised.

Hospital and patients

Over the last 30 years the rates of hospital admission have increased, despite the reduction in the number of beds. This has been achieved by decreasing the length of stay in hospital of each patient; for example

in 1984, repair of a groin hernia necessitated a stay of 4.9 days. It is now commonly done as day surgery.

When patients are admitted to hospital, they may find themselves disempowered by the experience. Medical staff, by virtue of their technical expertise, good health and familiarity with the practices on the wards, are in a considerable position of power and authority over the patients. The experience is commonly a source of anxiety and stress. The reasons for this may be due to the following:

1. The fact that there is 'something wrong' with them that has necessitated their admission.
2. A lack of privacy on the wards.
3. A lack of familiarity.
4. Being disturbed (by other patients and staff).
5. Lack of sleep.
6. Lack of information about their health.
7. Uncertainty about the process of care, procedures on the ward and which investigations will be necessary.
8. Uncertainty about the pain and risk involved in investigations and treatment.

9. What to expect post surgery – how long they will have to stay in hospital.
10. Concern about those at home.
11. Concern about employment and when they can get back to work.

Attempts to combat this negative experience include providing information about what to expect in hospital prior to admission. However, the experience of in-patient care gives rise not only to anxiety, but also to feelings of a *depersonalization* or loss of self identity. This is due to:

- A loss of normal social roles.
- The sense of being part of a 'batch' of patients being treated.
- The general impersonal nature of medical procedures.
- An institutionalized schedule – being told when to eat, when to get up, when visitors are allowed.
- A lack of privacy and personal possessions.

Patients who remain in hospital for long periods of time may be at risk of *institutionalization* (this was relatively common in long-stay psychiatric hospitals – and was one of the reasons for the development of the care in the community ethos).

Institutionalization refers to the process by which patients in 'total institutions' (those where individuals are wholly separated from social interaction with the outside world, e.g. old-style psychiatric hospitals, monasteries and prisons) become apathetic and unable to make simple decisions for themselves.

The psychological well-being of patients also impacts on their physical illness. If patients become anxious, stressed or depersonalized whilst in hospital, there is a real risk that their recovery from their physical illness will be slowed. Patients' beliefs about their illness seem to influence recovery and rehabilitation on discharge from hospital: one study showed that the early identification of illness perception could improve patient outcome following a myocardial infarction.

Chronic disease

Chronic disease has been identified as an increasing problem for modern medicine. This is partly due to the ageing population, but also due to the success of medicine in averting death, but not always avoiding permanent injury. Chronic disease often requires a 'caring' approach rather than a 'curative' one. By its very nature, chronic disease is a long-term affliction, and as such has a profound influence on those who suffer with it. Chronic diseases include arthritis, heart disease, some forms of cancer, ulcerative colitis, psoriasis, dementia, multiple sclerosis, asthma and epilepsy. A chronic disease may or may not eventually be fatal, in fact the severity of many of the diseases mentioned fluctuates greatly, both between sufferers and between days (or even hours) for the same sufferer.

Chronic disease poses a problem for Parsons' 'sick role' (as previously mentioned in this chapter), which expects the sick to want to get better and to only occupy the sick role temporarily. For the chronically ill, the 'sick role' must be modified slightly. Sufferers must maximize their ability to carry out social roles within the confines of their illness, and only be accepted to the 'sick role' when their capabilities drop below what they are usually able to do.

Study of the 'experience' of those living with chronic disease and their families has been undertaken since the 1980s in order to bring about a 'sound, effective and ethical approach to chronic illness' (Anderson & Bury 1988). A few of the common problems experienced by the chronically ill and disabled are mentioned below (adapted from Locker 2003, p. 87):

- *Uncertainty* – chronic disease can be shrouded in uncertainty. Symptoms may be present for many years before a definitive diagnosis is given (for example in multiple sclerosis). However, being given a diagnosis doesn't end the uncertainty. Patients (and doctors) may be unsure of how a disease will progress and at what speed. In addition symptoms may vary from day to day, with little rhyme or reason. One such disease is rheumatoid arthritis – pain level may vary throughout the day, often without a precipitating factor. The uncertainty means it is difficult to make even short-term plans, and living arrangements may need to be constantly revised.
- *Strained family relations* – often family members become carers for those who are chronically ill. The ability of individuals to cope with their role is varied and the carer (as well as the sufferer) may find themselves being excluded from their wider social contacts. Strain may also be placed on marital relationships. In a study of the effects of having a colostomy post rectal cancer, most individuals reported a loss of sexual capacity and a decline in the marital relationship.

- *Problems relating to self-esteem and identity* – the development of a chronic disease can lead to a fundamental rethinking of a person's biography and self-concept (Lawton 2003). This has been termed 'biographical disruption' by Bury (1982). Bury argues that such disruption can take place on many levels – including physical discomfort as well as a rethinking on one's mortality and existential sense. Charmaz (1983) outlined a similar perspective that describes a profound effect on the sense of self-worth, referred to as a 'loss of self', where individuals separate off the person they may have become as the disease progresses from a cherished view of how they were prior to the disability. Subsequent to the disruption and loss of an earlier conception of oneself comes the rebuilding of one's identity, which incorporates the chronic disease. Williams (1984) refers to this as 'narrative reconstruction'. This describes the strategies people employ 'to create a sense of coherence, stability and order in the aftermath of the "biographically disruptive" event of illness onset'. The view of oneself may become linked almost exclusively with that of the disease – to the exclusion of other social roles – so, a patient with multiple sclerosis views themselves as 'an MS sufferer' rather than a mother, a teacher, a theatre-goer or any other role she plays.
- *Problems relating to medical regimes* – patients with chronic diseases need to manage both their symptoms and their medical treatments on a daily basis. Often the treatment may be complicated – for example patients in renal failure who have dialysis – and time-consuming. Everyday life must be centred around the routine of medical treatment. This may prevent spontaneity and flexibility within the lifestyles of the chronically ill.
- *Unemployment and economic problems* – the most vulnerable groups in the face of chronic illness are those from low socioeconomic groups, ethnic minorities and women. Lower amounts of disposable income mean that individuals have fewer resources to support themselves through their disease. However, employment is important for reasons beyond simple economic benefit. Being able to be employed is significant in giving purpose and a focus for individuals and being 'included' in a social role may provide valuable benefits in terms of self-esteem.
- *Information, awareness and sharing* – information is a significant resource for the chronically ill. This may be about the disease from which they suffer, about the benefits they are entitled to, or coping strategies, or potential symptomatic treatments. The arena where such information sharing may occur is often a self-help group. The ability to meet others with the same disorder, and similar experiences, may also be beneficial (see p. 83).
- *Stigma and discrimination* – discussed above (pp. 88–89).

Chronic illness legislation
In 1970 the Chronically Sick and Disabled Persons Act was passed. This obliged local authorities to identify people with disabilities, determine their needs and provide appropriate services to meet those needs.

Living with chronic illness

The ability to adapt to living with a chronic illness can be divided into three different components:

1. *Coping* – the cognitive processes of learning how to tolerate or put up with the effects of illness.
2. *Strategies* – the actions people take, or what people do in the face of illness.
3. *Style* – the way people respond to and present important features of their illnesses or treatment regimen.

Factors that may aid individuals with chronic disease include (Verbrugge & Jette 1994):

- Extra-individual factors:
  - medical care and rehabilitation – surgery, physical therapy, speech therapy, counselling, health education, job retraining, etc.
  - medication and other therapeutic regimens – drugs, recreational therapy, aquatic exercise, biofeedback meditation, rest/energy conservation, etc.
  - external supports – personal assistance, special equipment and devices, day care, respite care, meals-on-wheels, etc.
  - build, physical and social environment – structural modifications at home or work, access

to buildings and public transport, health insurance and access to medical care, laws and regulations, employment legislation, social attitudes, etc.

- Intra-individual factors:
  – lifestyle and behaviour changes – overt changes to alter disease activity and impact
  – psychosocial attributes and coping – positive affect, emotional vigour, locus of control, cognitive adaptation to disability, personal support, peer support groups, etc.
  – activity accommodations – changes in kinds of activities, ways of doing them, frequency or length of time doing them.

Impairment, disability, handicap and the 'social model of disability'

Chronic disease is often associated with a degree of impairment in functioning. How this relates to terms like disability and handicap is set out by the International Classification of Impairments, Disabilities and Handicaps (ICIDH).

Crucial to the ICIDH definitions is the idea that handicaps are disadvantages that are not inherent in

International Classification of Impairments, Disabilities and Handicaps (ICIDH) definitions

- Impairment: any loss or abnormality of psychological, physiological or anatomical structure or function, e.g. osteoarthritis causing painful, stiff joints.
- Disability: a restriction or lack (resulting from an impairment) of ability to perform an activity in a manner or within the range considered normal for a human being, e.g. difficulty climbing stairs.
- Handicap: a disadvantage for a given individual, resulting from an impairment or a disability, that limits or prevents the fulfilment of a role that is normal (depending on age, sex and social and cultural factors) for that individual, e.g. an inability to access certain buildings within the community with steps – thus perhaps being unable to visit certain cinemas, libraries, banks and so on.

the individuals, rather they are imposed by the environment. However, the ICIDH definitions have been criticized for using the term 'handicap', which to many is considered a pejorative term.

Disability campaigners over the past 20 years have advocated a theory known as the 'social model of disability'. This approach stands in contrast to the 'medical model of disability', which sees disabilities and handicaps as directly and inevitably derived from impairments.

The social model of disability states that:

- Disabled people are an oppressed social group.
- There is a difference between the impairments people have and the oppression they experience.
- 'Disability' can be defined as the social oppression, not the form of impairment.

This model describes disability as something imposed upon those with impairments by unnecessarily isolating and excluding them from full participation in society. Disability is the 'social situation' encountered by people with impairments. The importance of this model is twofold:

1. It identifies the proper approach to disability as being the removal of those barriers that prevent people with impairments from fully participating in society, rather than the previous medicalized approach, which was to cure and 'normalize' impairments.
2. It liberates and empowers the disabled community by locating fault with society rather than with disabled individuals.

However, the social model of disability has been criticized on the following grounds:

1. The denial of the link between physical impairment and social disability has been overstated – denying that disabled people are not also people with impairments is to ignore a major part of the biographies of disabled people.
2. Emphasis on criticizing the need for a 'cure', as stated by the medical model, has led to some disabled groups opposing measures designed to 'normalise' their conditions or maximise their function. For example, the refusal of artificial limbs for amputees and hearing aids for the hearing impaired. This has led to certain conditions having a greater impact on people's lives than might otherwise have been the case.
3. The social model is too rigid in creating an artificial distinction between disability and impairment – the two can be seen as part of a continuum.

4. Some impairments cannot be helped by the removal of environmental or social barriers (e.g. phantom limb pain and significant intellectual impairment).

Disability legislation
In 1995 the Disability Discrimination Act was passed, which begins to address many of the social issues identified in the social model of disability. See www.disability.gov.uk

Death and bereavement

The way in which death is perceived is determined by personal and cultural factors. In an increasingly secular culture, death is seen as a finality, beyond which there is no existence. However, many religions agree in some sort of afterlife, be it reincarnation or a spiritual paradise. In some traditional societies it is believed that the dead do not really die, at least not in a social sense, rather they remain as an invisible spirit that is still a member of the family and can help, protect, hinder or punish those who continue to survive in an earthly way.

Our perception of death changes as we age. Young children see death as a sleep or departure, not understanding the finality of death until about the age of seven. Children are at first matter of fact and then fearful of corpses. The perception and understanding of death within Western culture is one that tends to incorporate feelings of loss, separation, pain and punishment.

One hundred years ago, less than 10% of people died in hospitals. It is thought that about 75% of people now die (in the UK) in institutions such as hospitals, hospices and nursing homes. The general trend has been for death and the process of dying to be removed from the public domain. Part of the reason for this is the greater ability of medical technology to prolong life; as a result the process of dying is more drawn out, leading to 'slow deaths'. Figure 5.7 compares slow dying in the modern era with 'quick deaths' in the pre-modern era.

The stages of dying

The typical stages of dying were described in 1969 by Elizabeth Kubler-Ross, an American psychiatrist:

1. Denial and isolation: on being told they are dying patients may enter a state of shock, expressing feelings like 'It can't be me'. Denial is usually a temporary defence, although it can be sustained. Patients may 'shop around' for a more positive second opinion. A deep feeling of isolation is 'normal' at this stage.
2. Anger: shock may be replaced by feelings of anger, resentment and rage. The medical staff – often the nurses – may be subjected to outbursts of 'Why me?' and 'Why can't you help me?'
3. Bargaining: the terminally ill may attempt to negotiate with care givers, or God. They may

Fig. 5.7 A comparison of death and the process of dying in the 'modern' and 'pre-modern' eras.

A comparison of death and the process of dying in the 'modern' and 'pre-modern' eras	
Conditions facilitating a 'quick death'	**Conditions facilitating a 'slow death'**
Low level of medical technology	High level of medical technology
Late detection of disease – or fatality-producing condition	Early detection of disease – or fatality-producing condition
Simple definition of death (e.g. cessation of heart beat)	Complex definition of death (e.g. irreversible cessation of higher brain activity)
High incidence of mortality from acute disease	High incidence of mortality from chronic or degenerative disease
High incidence of fatality-producing injuries	Low incidence of fatality-producing injuries
Customary killing or suicide of, or fatal passivity towards, the person once he or she has entered the 'dying' category	Customary curative and activist orientation toward the dying with a high value placed on the prolongation of life

Source: Lofland L 1978 The Craft of Dying: the Modern Face of Death. Beverly Hills: Sage Publications; as reprinted in Scambler G 2003 Dying, death and bereavement. In: Scambler G (ed.) Sociology as Applied to Medicine, 5th edn. Edinburgh: Saunders, p. 93

endeavour to be a 'good' patient in order that the doctor might extend their lives.

4. Depression: as patients confront their fate, their anger or shock may give way to depression, it may be reactive – to the condition, or preparatory – based on the impending loss of life itself.

5. Acceptance: dying patients may find a sort of peace, an acknowledgement of the inevitability of death. At this stage the family may need more help, support and understanding than the patient.

Kubler-Ross' model rapidly gained acceptance, according to some, because it filled a void in health-care theory and re-awakened the topic of dying that had previously been taboo. However, it was criticized because:

- It assumed too mechanistic an approach, with the dying person moving through all five stages in one direction, whilst the experience of those caring for the dying suggested an oscillation between periods of calm, fear, hope, depression, anger and withdrawal.
- It focused on psychological aspects of dying, at the expense of physical and spiritual dimensions.

Subsequent authors have modified the stages model of dying by increasing the mixture of emotions and responses exhibited by a person facing death (Fig. 5.8) and marking a patient's progress by the resolution of these emotions, rather than their change. However, this model still suffers from the criticism that it focuses only on the psychological aspects of dying.

Corr (1992) developed a theory that states that individuals who are dying confront tasks in four dimensions of coping with death. These are:

- Physical – satisfying bodily needs – such as thirst and pain.
- Psychological – this includes maximizing psychological security and autonomy.
- Social – this includes sustaining and enhancing interpersonal attachments of significance to the person, and addressing the social implications of dying; for example, wanting to know that dependants will be cared for after their death.
- Spiritual – for many people, identifying and reaffirming a sense of spirituality may foster hope or bring reassurance.

Corr maintained that individuals have unique circumstances leading to unique tasks they must cope with in each of these dimensions. The advantage of this model of dying is that it encompasses different aspects of the process rather than focusing on the psychological aspect alone. However, its generality and lack of empirical data limit its usefulness.

The Debate of the Age Health and Care Study Group (1999) produced the following principles necessary for a 'good death':

- To know when death is coming, and to understand what can be expected.
- To be able to retain control of what happens.
- To be afforded dignity and privacy.
- To have control over pain relief and also symptom control.

Fig. 5.8 Three-stage model of dying.

Three-stage model of dying

Initial stage 'facing the threat'	Chronic stage 'being ill'	Final stage 'acceptance'
Fear	Resolution of those elements of the initial response that are resolvable	Defined by patient's acceptance of death
Anxiety		
Shock	Diminution of intensity of all emotions	Not an essential state provided that the patient is not distressed, is communicating normally and is making decisions normally
Disbelief		
Anger	Depression	
Denial		
Guilt		
Humour		
Hope		
Despair		
Bargaining		

Source: Buckman R 1993 Communication in palliative care: a practical guide. In: Doyle D, Hanks GWC, McDonald N (eds) Oxford Textbook of Palliative Medicine. Oxford: Oxford Medical Publications

- To have choice and control over where death occurs (at home or elsewhere).
- To have access to information and expertise of whatever kind is necessary.
- To have access to any spiritual or emotional support required.
- To have access to hospice care in any location, not only in hospital.
- To have control over who is present and who shares the end.
- To be able to issue advance directives that ensure wishes are respected.
- To have time to say goodbye, and control over other aspects of timing.
- To be able to leave when it is time to go, and not to have life prolonged pointlessly.

Place of death

As mentioned earlier, over the past 100 years there has been an increasing trend in dying outside the home. This has led to a situation where most people die in hospitals or other institutions. Each location has certain advantages and disadvantages associated with it.

Dying at home

To many the home remains the proper and natural place to die. Dying at home may be more costly and physically and emotionally demanding for carers. For this reason it requires good communication between hospital services and the carers. Additional support, in the form of respite care, meals on wheels, and Macmillan nurses may be welcomed.

Dying in a hospice

This accounts for around only 4% of deaths. The hospice philosophy is one that concentrates on promoting quality of life over prolonging life. Dying in a hospice may bring reduced levels of anxiety and depression when compared to similar care in hospitals – this may be due to a culture of frank and honest communication.

Dying in hospitals

Hospitals have not historically been especially quick to have wards dedicated solely to the treatment of the terminally ill, fearing the stigma that may be attached to such 'death wards'. However, this has led to some terminally ill patients dying on busy general wards, which is unsatisfactory to all patients, families and staff concerned. One study has demonstrated that many patients' symptoms are not adequately controlled, and many received inadequate nursing care. Furthermore, terminally ill patients may receive only minimal care from senior medical and nursing staff on general wards.

Dying in retirement villages

In North America, retirement villages have been set up and some have been associated with specialist nursing facilities that are available to those requiring terminal care. This sort of facility has allowed elderly residents to talk amongst themselves about death, and has enabled a shared perspective and collective concern to develop. Residents feel a greater degree of control over the process of dying. It differs from traditional nursing homes where the dying person is isolated from other residents.

Awareness of dying

Glaser and Strauss (1965) described four different types of 'awareness context' in the management of dying patients in San Francisco Bay area hospitals in the 1960s. These were:

1. *Closed awareness*: where patients were kept ignorant of their impending death by staff and family alike.
2. *Suspicion awareness*: where patients had begun to suspect that they were dying and had tried to obtain confirmation of this suspicion from both staff and relatives.
3. *Mutual pretence*: where all parties knew that that the patient was dying, but no-one acknowledged this fact.
4. *Open awareness*: where all parties knew that the patient was dying and were able to talk about dying.

Since the 1960s there has been a progressive move away from the closed awareness context towards one of open awareness. Open awareness is now seen as a prerequisite for a 'good death'. There is a general consensus that honesty within the medical consultation is necessary even when the patient has a terminal disease.

Outcomes of open awareness

For the patient:
- Better information and communication from staff.
- Psychological support.
- Participation in decisions about care.
- Increased self-esteem.
- Decreased anxiety.
- Preparation for death.
- Acceptance.

For relatives/carers:
- More honest relationship with the patient.
- Easier communication with patient and staff.
- Better bereavement outcomes.

For the doctors and nurses:
- Easier interaction with the patient.
- Shared decision-making.
- Less anxiety, guilt, stress that accompany deceiving the patient.
- Being able to stop inappropriate treatments.

In the past decade or so the concept of *conditional open awareness* has developed. This stresses that disclosure can take place over a period of time and that full disclosure of terminal prognoses is conditional on what is desirable for particular patients. Some individuals may not wish to discuss their terminal prognosis. Conditional open awareness is characterized by a shared approach to confronting death, or if the patient wishes to do so, denying a terminal prognosis. The aim is to act in such a way as to produce a positive psychological outcome for the patient.

Bereavement and loss

One-quarter of GP consultations have been identified as relating to some type of loss – these include separations, incapacitation, bereavement, and job losses. Any loss can lead to a detrimental effect on physical and mental health. A major bereavement, such as the death of a spouse or child, can increase the risk of death from heart disease and suicide as well as increasing the likelihood of anxiety and depression.

Even though mourning can be expressed in a variety of ways there is still a pattern to grieving, and it can make sense to talk of a 'normal pattern of grief'. Worden (1991) outlines a number of tasks that need to be achieved in the course of mourning if it is to be completed:
- Task I: To accept the reality of the loss:
  - The bereaved is initially shocked, and may experience numbness, disbelief or relief at the death.

Bereavement and patterns of expressed grief
The pattern of mourning varies from community to community. For some Greek-Cypriots there is a 'socially patterned period of weeping and wailing' followed by a defined period of mourning and wearing black. In Orthodox Jewish communities there is a prescribed timetable to mourning – in the first seven days, the bereaved remain at home and are visited by consolers. Mourning dress is worn for 30 days, and recreation and amusement are forbidden for one year.

- Task II: To work through the pain of grief:
  - The bereaved may experience anger, sadness, guilt, anxiety, regret, insomnia and even transient auditory or visual hallucinations of the deceased.
- Task III: To adjust to an environment in which the deceased is missing:
  - This may be characterized by despair and a loss of direction. The bereaved may perceive themselves as helpless, inadequate and childlike.
- Task IV: To emotionally relocate the deceased and move on with life:
  - During this phase, the bereaved may start to develop new relationships and interests. The deceased is no longer central in the bereaved person's emotional life.

There is evidence that losses can help to foster maturity and personal growth; however, there are a number of factors that are associated with a poor outcome (Fig. 5.9).

Fig. 5.9 Risk factors for poor outcome of bereavement.

Risk factors for poor outcome of bereavement

Predisposing factors

Ambivalent or dependent relationship with the person who died
Multiple prior bereavements
Previous mental illness, especially depression
Low self-esteem of bereaved person
Age and sex of bereaved person – older widowers are at greater risk than widows and younger individuals. Similarly the death of a parent is associated with greater risk if the bereaved person is still a child or adolescent, as opposed to an older individual, with their own family

Around the time of death

Sudden and unexpected death
Untimely death of a young person
Deaths due to suicide/murder/manslaughter
Stigmatized death: such as AIDS

After death

Level of perceived social support – for example an absent or unhelpful family
Lack of opportunities for new interests
Stress from other life crises

Source: Based on Sheldon 1998 ABC of Palliative Care: Bereavement. British Medical Journal 316: 456–58

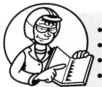

- Define illness, disease, sickness and predicaments.
- What factors are important in the evaluation of symptoms?
- What is the function of self-help groups?
- Why do you think use of alternative medicine has been increasing?
- What is the 'sick role'?
- What is 'labelling'?
- What characterizes a 'patient-centred consultation'?
- How can communication skills be improved?
- Define compliance and concordance.
- Why is hospital admission associated with anxiety and stress?
- What sorts of problems are experienced by people with chronic illness?
- How do impairment, disability and handicap differ?
- What is the 'social model of disability'?
- What are the 'stages of dying'?

References

Alonzo A, Reynolds N 1995 Stigma, HIV and AIDS: an exploration and elaboration of a stigma strategy. Social Sciences in Medicine 41:303–15

Anderson R, Bury M (eds) 1988 as quoted by Locker D, Living with chronic illness. In: Scambler G (ed) 2003 Sociology as Applied to Medicine, 5th edn. Edinburgh: Saunders, p. 79

Armstrong D 1989 An Outline of Sociology as Applied to Medicine, 3rd edn. London: Wright

Banks MH, Beresford SA, Morrell D et al. 1975 Factors influencing demand for primary medical care in women aged 20–44. International Journal of Epidemiology 4: 189–95, as reproduced in Armstrong D 1989 An Outline of Sociology as Applied to Medicine, 3rd edn. London: Wright

Blaxter M 1990 Health and Lifestyles. London: Tavistock/Routledge

Boorse C 1975 On the distinction between disease and illness. Philosophy and Public Affairs 5: 49–68

Boorse C 1976 What a theory of mental health should be. Journal for the Theory of Social Behaviour 6: 61–85

Britten N et al. 2000 Misunderstandings in prescribing decisions in general practice: qualitative study. British Medical Journal 320: 484–88

Bury M 1982 Chronic illness as biographical disruption. Sociology of Health & Illness 4: 167–82

Charmaz K 1983 Loss of self: a fundamental form of suffering in the chronically ill. Sociology of Health and Illness 5: 168–95, as reported by Nettleton S 1995 The Sociology of Health and Illness. Cambridge: Polity Press p. 87

Corr CA 1992 A task based approach to coping with dying. Omega 24(2) 81–94, as reproduced in Copp G 1998 A review of current theories of death and dying. Journal of Advanced Nursing 28(2): 382–90

Cox K et al. 2003 A systematic review of communication between patients and health care professionals about medicine-taking and prescribing. London: GKT Concordance Unit, King's College, as quoted in Weiss M, Britten N 2003 What is concordance? The Pharmaceutical Journal 271:493

Damen S, Mortelmans D, Hove E 2000 Self-help groups in Belgium: their place in the care network. Sociology of Health & Illness 22(3): 331–48

Debate of the Age Health and Care Study Group 1999 The Future of Health and Care of Older People: The best is yet to come. London: Age Concern

Glaser B, Strauss A 1965 Awareness of Dying. Chicago: Aldine

Goffman E 1963 Stigma: Notes on the Management of Spoiled Identity. London: Penguin

Hannay D 1988 Lecture Notes on Medical Sociology. Oxford: Blackwell Scientific Publications, p. 138

Kubler-Ross E 1969 On Death and Dying. New York: Macmillan

Lawton J 2003 Lay experiences of health and illness: past research and future agendas. Sociology of Health & Illness 25: 26–27

Locker D 2003 Living with chronic illness. In: Scambler G (ed.) Sociology as Applied to Medicine, 5th edn. Edinburgh: Saunders, pp. 79–91

Mead N, Bower P 2002 Patient-centred consultations and outcomes in primary care: a review of the literature. Patient Education and Counseling 48: 51–61

Mechanic D 1978 Medical Sociology. New York: The Free Press

Mechanic D, Volkart EH 1960 Illness behaviour and medical diagnosis. Journal of Health and Human Behaviour 1: 86–94

Medicines Partnership What is concordance? Available online at http://www.medicines-partnership.org/about-us/concordance

Morgan M 2003 The doctor–patient relationship. In: Scambler G (ed.) Sociology as Applied to Medicine, 5th edn. Edinburgh: Saunders, p. 49

Parsons T 1951 The Social System. Glencoe, IL: Free Press, as quoted by Morgan M in: Scambler G (ed.) 2003 Sociology as Applied to Medicine, 5th edn. Edinburgh: Saunders, p. 51

Roter D 2000 The enduring and evolving nature of the patient–physician relationship. Patient Education and Counseling 39(5–15): 8

Royal Pharmaceutical Society of Great Britain 1997 From compliance to concordance: towards shared goals in medicine taking. London: RPS

Scambler G 2003 Deviance, sick role and stigma. In Scambler G (ed.) Sociology as Applied to Medicine, 5th edn. Edinburgh: Saunders, pp. 192–202

Scambler G, Hopkins A 1986 Being epileptic: coming to terms with stigma. Sociology of Health and Illness 8: 26–43, as reported in Scambler G 2003 Deviance, sick role and stigma. In: Scambler G (ed.) 2003 Sociology as Applied to Medicine, 5th edn. Edinburgh: Saunders, p. 196

Toon PD 1981 Defining 'disease' – classification must be distinguished from evaluation. Journal of Medical Ethics 7: 197–201

Towle A, Godolphin W 1999 Framework for teaching and learning informed shared decision making. British Medical Journal 319: 766–71

Verbrugge LM, Jette AM 1994 The disablement process. Social Science and Medicine 38: 1–14, as reproduced in Locker D 1997 Living with chronic illness. In Scambler D (ed.) An Outline of Sociology as Applied to Medicine. Edinburgh: Saunders, p. 78

Williams G 1984 The genesis of chronic illness: narrative reconstruction. Sociology of Health and Illness 6: 175–200

Worden JW 1991 Grief Counselling and Grief Therapy. London: Routledge, pp. 7–21

Zborowski M 1952 Cultural components in response to pain. Journal of Social Issues 8: 16–30

Zola I 1973 Pathways to the doctor: from person to patient. Social Science and Medicine 7: 677–889, as reported in Scambler G 2003 Health and illness behaviour. In Scambler G (ed.) Sociology as Applied to Medicine, 5th edn. Edinburgh: Saunders

Further reading

Barry C et al. 2000 Patients' unvoiced agendas in general practice consultations: qualitative study. British Medical Journal 320: 1246–50

Scambler G (ed.) 2003 Sociology as Applied to Medicine, 5th edn. Edinburgh: Saunders

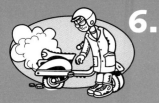

6. Organization of Health-care Provision in the UK

Before the NHS

From the 19th century to the mid-20th century several asynchronous components of the health-care system attempted to provide the best possible treatment for the patient:

- General practitioners (GPs) – mainly for those who could afford them, were part of insurance schemes, e.g. the Friendly Societies (non-profit-making, mutual benefit organizations), or were affiliated with trade unions.
- Hospitals – primarily used by the poor. They were either *voluntary* (run by charitable foundations) or *municipal* (local authority) hospitals. The latter provided services to the poorest of people and the unemployed.
- Public health and community health services (CHS) – aimed to improve the water supplies and sewerage; eventually, they attempted to control and treat infectious diseases. Public health, CHS (and housing) were under the control of the local authorities, not health services, and this continued until the early 1970s.

Another crucial aspect to remember is that, in the 19th century, hospitals were considered very dangerous places owing to the lack of anaesthesia and aseptic techniques. For those who could afford it, a fee-for-service consultation with a qualified practitioner in the surgery or at home was possible. Friendly Societies, which were non-profit-making and mutual-benefit organizations and trade unions allowed other groups, e.g. skilled workers, to use GPs.

The same era also saw the *Poor Law* system being practised. This catered for the needs of the very poorest people and the unemployed. However, patients had to be 'deservingly poor' to qualify for treatment. Even though the standards of these hospitals rose in the 1930s when they were taken on by local authority health departments, their status always remained low owing to their origins.

The introduction of the NHS was one of the greatest of public health initiatives.

The birth of the NHS

During World War II, it emerged that the state could have a positive impact on the lives of its people by improving their well-being. Also, all hospitals had been brought under state control as part of the Emergency Medical Service. The famous Beveridge Report (1942) established the principles for a post-war 'welfare state'. In 1944, the Ministry of Health set out its plans for a comprehensive health service. After a series of negotiations between the government and the British Medical Association (BMA), the National Health Service Act (1946) came into being. In 1948, the NHS was born (Fig. 6.1).

Interestingly, the financial estimates that were put to Parliament along with the White Paper setting up the NHS anticipated a fall in the cost of the NHS based on the assumptions of effective health promotion and improved public health leading to improved health of the population.

Evolution

The NHS has proved to be a fairly dynamic system undergoing continuous reform, particularly since the

---

Key features of the NHS

- Free at the point of use
- Open to the whole population purely on the basis of health-care need
- Equality in provision of health services irrespective of means, age, sex and occupation
- Funded almost entirely by general taxation revenues collected by the government

Fig. 6.1 Key features of the NHS.

Chronological list of landmark events in the shaping of the NHS

Period	Problems	Solutions
1948–74	Divisions between GPs, local authority health services and teaching hospitals	More integrated structure with regional health authorities overseeing area health authorities so correct dispatch of finances to hospitals and community health services
	Inequalities in the geographical distribution of hospital beds and staff requirements	GPs remained independent
	Rising expenditure relative to conservative estimates	*Hospital plan for England and Wales* proposed the creation of a modern district general hospital (DGH) that could treat 250 000 people
		Charges introduced for spectacles, dentures and prescriptions
1982–87	Difficult for central government to set policy, oversee expenditure and monitor performance	Single general manager appointed at every level in the NHS with power to undertake executive decisions over the resources they managed
		Quantitative performance indicators (PIs) introduced
1988	Demand greater than supply	Increased general taxation
	Inadequate funding resulting in poor maintenance of infrastructure, low staff pay and lowering standard of care	
	Increasing waiting lists	
1989–90	Funding crisis continues	*Community Care Act* (1990) became law. Internal market introduced to separate the roles of purchaser and provider
		New GP contract giving autonomy to larger GP practices. Medical audit made compulsory for both hospitals and GPs. Health authorities streamlined. Increase in the number of managers to increase efficiency
1991–97	Poor implementation of internal market	'New Labour' elected in 1997 – tried to find an intermediate ground between market forces and socialism
	Too much control by central government	
1997–2000	Too much emphasis on *quantity* rather than *quality* of health care	A new system based on 'partnership' and 'collaboration'
	Internal market getting chaotic	Regional autonomy – separate White Papers introduced for England, Ireland, Wales and Scotland
		Individual funding for GP practices abolished, instead they got their funding from their local Primary Care Group (PCG) or Primary Care Trust (PCT)
		National Institute for Clinical Excellence (NICE) set up in 1999 to assess the best available evidence on the effectiveness and cost-effectiveness of treatments, drugs and technologies (old and new) and to produce official guidance on whether they should be funded as part of the NHS
		Commission for Health Improvement (CHI) set up in 2000 to monitor and improve the quality of NHS services
2000–present	Lack of modernization. Waiting lists increasing. Varying public confidence	Making the NHS more receptive to the needs of its users. Establishment of NHS Direct and NHS walk-in centres. Setting NHS plan performance targets. Public–private partnerships encouraged. PCTs are expected to control 75% of the NHS budget by 2004

Fig. 6.2 Chronological list of landmark events in the shaping of the NHS.

108

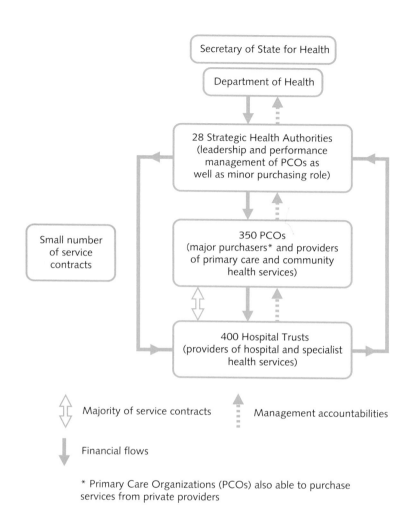

1970s. Its ultimate goal has always been to improve the quality of patient care.

Its changes can be divided into *three* phases:

1. *Hierarchical (1948–79)* – totalitarian control by officials and politicians at a national level. A classic example of 'top-down' regulation.
2. *Market (1979–97)* – introduction of market mechanism, dividing purchasers from providers and encouraging the competitive tendering of support services, e.g. cleaning.
3. *Network (1997–present)* – amalgamating the pros and cons of (a) and (b) above. Encouraging

collaborations and partnerships within the system (Fig. 6.2).

Current organization

This chapter is based on the organization of the NHS in England. There are variations in other areas of the UK. The organization of the NHS is based on giving the primary care organizations (PCOs) greater freedom to make the purchasing decisions for local health services. All GPs are members of PCOs. It also strives to streamline the system overall whilst being user-friendly for the patient (Fig. 6.3).

The 21st century

The NHS has several strengths and weaknesses. These need to be understood so that as decision-makers of the future we know what areas to tackle (Fig. 6.4).

A major issue that will confront the NHS in the near future is the likely imbalance that will occur between health-care funding and usage.

It is estimated that one-third of all men aged between 50 and 65 years old do not work. This is due partly to early retirement and pension incentives or to employer-based age discrimination. Furthermore, the all-cause death rates have decreased in the last 20 years. People are living longer.

According to the government's own estimates, the number of people aged 65 years or older will double by the year 2036. NHS services to people in this age group account for a large proportion of NHS resources. As the total population is expected to remain stable, the proportion of older people will constitute 25% of the population.

Inevitably there will be increased spending by the government. However, the birth-rate has also been declining, meaning that there will be fewer young people entering the job market. If current trends continue, there will be a shortage of future tax-payers relative to the elderly. Other sources of finance will have to be sought apart from possible increases in general taxation.

↑ ageing population = ↑ strain on the NHS

Other systems for organizing and funding health care

Funding and provision of health care varies greatly in different countries. Over the course of the 20th century, governments have taken an active role in trying to provide the best possible health services.

Patients also have individual rights and expectations of their health-care system.

According to Fitzpatrick (2003), and Field (1973), health-care systems can be divided into four categories (Fig. 6.5):

1. The pluralistic health system, e.g. USA
   a. several non-integrated methods of providing funds, e.g. insurance, fee-for-service, etc.
   b. health-care facilities owned by private groups or the state.
2. The health insurance system, e.g. Canada, USA and Japan
   a. third party gathers resources in the form of compulsory insurance.
3. The health service system, e.g. UK and Sweden
   a. the state owns *most* facilities
   b. independence of doctors, despite the fact that they receive most of their income from the government.
4. The socialized health system, e.g. the former USSR
   a. the state owns *all* facilities
   b. nearly all health-care professionals are employed by the government.

Health professions

A vast number of professional groups provide health care in modern Britain. These include hospital doctors, nurses, radiographers, GPs, community nurses, care assistants, pharmacists and social workers, to name but a few. With so many professionals looking after the patient, there are bound to be problems, such as misunderstandings, poor communication, mistrust and sometimes conflict.

Clinical governance – current

According to the Department of Health, clinical governance is a framework through which the organizations that constitute the NHS are accountable for continuously improving the quality of their services and safeguarding high standards of care by creating an environment in which excellence in clinical care will flourish (Fig. 6.6).

At present, we need to understand why the quality of health care is variable. There is a need to provide a certain minimum standard of care for patients at all

Positives and negatives of the NHS today

Positives	Negatives
Wide public support	Lack of receptiveness to the needs of the patient coupled with lack of choice Professionals still regulate the service
Control of general spending whilst providing beneficial social programmes	Increased demand for greater spending Budget has not increased proportionately to demand or in line with other European countries
Good value for money	Fewer health-care professionals – doctors, nurses, etc.
Many services available with few user charges	Restricted access to latest drugs and technology
Services based on demand	Large discrepancy between quality and availability of specific services
General taxation provides finance	Parallel privately financed companies may compromise the fairness of the NHS in providing health care
Fair allocation of resources to different parts of the country	Interference by ministers in the fine details of health-care management
Excellent primary care via GPs	
Competent staff because of high-quality clinical training	
High degree of coordination	

Fig. 6.4 Positives and negatives of the NHS today.

Clinical governance can be simply defined as 'doing anything and everything required to maximize the quality of health-care provision'. Its aims are to:
- Promote clinical effectiveness through continuous facilitation.
- Weed out underperformance.
- Provide high-quality health-care services.

times. Furthermore, ways of reducing inequalities in sex, age, geography and ethnicity in the provision of health care need to be found.

The common areas prone to risk in providing health-care services are thought to be outdated clinical practice, poor communication and lack of continuity of care.

Clinical governance allows a coordinated approach to overcome the above areas of risk. It facilitates continuous development and encourages improvement.

There are major implications for all stakeholders in the NHS ranging from medical students and junior doctors to consultants. Some of these are the:
- Development of leadership and knowledge amongst clinicians.
- Development of mechanisms to ensure the 'audit loop' is closed, i.e. to ensure that change in clinical practice takes place in the *light of audit, research, evidence, risk management and complaints findings.*
- Development of appropriate accountability structures in both primary and secondary care.

Fig. 6.5 The advantages and disadvantages of different health-care systems.

The advantages and disadvantages of different health-care systems

System	Advantages	Disadvantages
Pluralistic	Closest to a market-driven system	Lack of access – many people cannot afford it Medical monopoly resulting in increased cost Individual access and lack of public-health initiatives
Health insurance	Easier access to private medical care Reduced waiting time Access to leading specialists	Insurance policies favour the use of cheaper medical procedures Premiums may vary according to age Not all medical procedures are covered by the policy
Health service	Universal access *Free* at point of use	Priority issues – continuous planning and changing of health-care provision Rationing – waiting lists bound to increase
Socialized	Everyone is equal and no other option, e.g. no private care for patients	Difficult to maintain quality and keep up with latest technologies Rationing Lack of responsiveness Risk of bribery as everyone is employed by the state

- Implementation of evidence-based practice across organizations.
- Improvement of the clinical information infrastructure of the NHS.
- Development of effective multi-disciplinary and inter-agency work.
- Integration of continuing medical education (CME) and continuing professional development (CPD) into quality-improvement programmes.

Health professions and multi-disciplinary working

The boundaries between doctors and nurses have changed. Nurses now take on prescribing and treatment roles. Also in the UK, the reduction in the number of working hours for junior doctors means that nurse practitioners have to take on some of the roles previously undertaken by doctors. There are several health-care professionals who look after the patient. There has been strong appreciation for the roles played by social workers, pharmacists, physiotherapists and nutritionists.

Carr-Saunders and Wilson (1933) defined 'professionals' according to their characteristics or traits:

- Possession of altruistic values – these are integral for functioning and performance is valued more than financial reward.
- High ethical standards.
- Discrete body of knowledge over which members have complete control.
- High social status.
- Monopoly position in market.
- Able to regulate their own working conditions independent of the state.

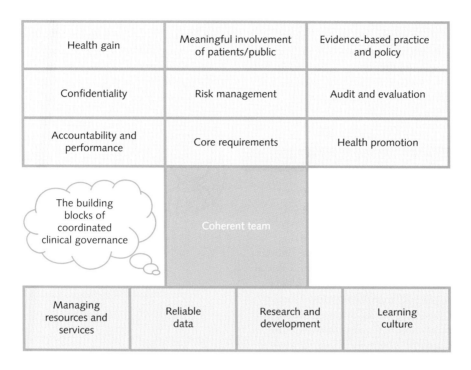

Health gain	Meaningful involvement of patients/public	Evidence-based practice and policy
Confidentiality	Risk management	Audit and evaluation
Accountability and performance	Core requirements	Health promotion

The building blocks of coordinated clinical governance

Coherent team

Managing resources and services	Reliable data	Research and development	Learning culture

Fig. 6.6 The 14 components of clinical governance.
Source: adapted from Chambers R, Booth E, Rogers D 2004 Stage 6 – what clinical governance means and how to put it into practise. In: Routes and branches of clinical governance, clinical effectiveness and clinical governance made easy. Oxford: Radcliffe Medical Press

- Lengthy period of training, the quality and content of which is determined by the profession itself.
- Striving to serve others.

While the 'trait-approach' has received criticism, it does serve to highlight the independence and power of some professional groups, particularly doctors. Larson (1977) introduces the idea of a 'professional project', which entails developing claims to a privileged social position and the ability to sustain this over time. MacDonald (1995) argues that professionals attempt to build up assets or capital in three ways:

1. *Economic assets* – including prestigious properties owned by The Royal Colleges.
2. *Organizational status* – health-care professionals are given power by the state to control large-scale organizations, e.g. the NHS.
3. *Cultural assets* – adequate scientific knowledge, reputation and credentials supported by the

activities of the professional bodies, e.g. the Royal Colleges, allow members to be key advisors to the government.

In general, the medical profession accumulated a lot of power up to the middle of the 20th century. This was due to its relationship with the state, the concept of a 'close-knit' group and the ability to dominate other groups.

Professional groups are under continuous scrutiny by the government, the public and the media. The entire medical profession has been shaken by high-profile cases of medical negligence and malpractice.

Clinical governance – history

During the 18th century, 22 different licensing bodies allowed individuals to practise medicine. Problems arose between the different groups of practitioners (which included apothecaries, physicians and surgeons), all of whom wanted the right to control newly founded hospitals as this allowed them to regulate 'official' health-care provision.

In 1858, the *Medical Registration Act* was passed and this led to the inception of the General Medical Council (GMC). Doctors were now united into a single group and this allowed the state to further its involvement in health care.

The holistic model

A holistic model of care involves all aspects of patient needs being addressed. The services provided by social workers, physiotherapists, pharmacists, nutritionists and occupational therapists are all important in providing a 'holistic' model of care for the patient. Some of the roles of the doctor are now performed by nurses. These include prescribing and treatment roles. There is also a move to have surgical assistants who are experienced nurses and have undergone further training to perform simple procedures, thereby giving the surgeons time to deal with the complicated cases.

Care in the community

The term 'community care' describes how society should meet the health and social needs of dependent people – specifically, care in the community (i.e. not in hospital) by the community (i.e. by carers/community health-care practitioners). It also refers to the services that are currently provided to dependent groups.

Dependent groups include the:
- Elderly.
- Chronically ill.
- People with disabilities.

Since the 1980s, informal care from family, friends, relatives and voluntary organizations has become more significant and public as the shift from institutional care to community care has been enacted. The key obstacles to implementation of effective community care are a lack of resources, managerial difficulties and coordination between social and health services. All health-care professionals should acknowledge the rise of carers and provide them with sufficient information and support to both help the person they care for and help themselves.

The *NHS and Community Care Act 1990* dictates the working together of local authority social services and the NHS, so as to harmonize packages of care with other agencies and users. Subsequent legislation requires these services also to take account of the needs of informal carers.

The fundamental driving forces for community care are:
- Reduction in hospital beds – their number has been diminishing for a long time partly due to improvement in techniques and policies that allow short stays in hospital, and also to reduce costs. There has also been an increase in the use of day surgery and reduced stay for acute medical conditions.
- Patient and client groups – all patients can benefit from good community care. In particular, dependent groups can be treated more effectively in this manner and reduce the time spent at institutions, e.g. hospitals (Fig. 6.7).

Community care can to a certain extent be funded by the reduced costs brought about by the closure of bigger institutions, but sufficient bridging funding must be established so that appropriate community care is set up prior to discharging people from bigger institutions.

Setting up effective community health-care initiatives has several hurdles:
- *Political accountability* – the government determines the health-care system that a nation adopts and as such decides how much funding it gets.

Why move to community care?	
Factor	**Explanation**
Demographic	An ageing population is safer under community care
Economic	Value for money, flexibility of community services and minimal fixed costs
Technological	More can be done at home by the GP and community nurses
Consumer choice	The general feeling is that it is user-friendly

Fig. 6.7 Why move to community care?

- *Diversity* – how many services can the organization provide, e.g. podiatry, psychiatry, community nursing, etc.
- *Complex and rapidly changing external environment* – economic, sociological, technological and political factors will determine which health policies are rapidly initiated.
- *Changing technologies* – unlike hospitals, which have the latest technology, human skills in community-care settings have been taken for granted and it is only recently that the latter has benefited from advances in information technology.
- *Working conditions* – stakeholders in community care need to recognize the factors that motivate their health professionals and support staff.

Current problems

There is still a shortage of community-care places, especially for elderly people as well as those with learning disabilities and mental illness. In addition, these groups use the health service more often than other groups. Given the diversity and increased need among inner-city inhabitants, especially the homeless and refugees, it seems that community care could go a long way in providing effective health care for these groups. Primary care needs to be reformed to give equal importance to community health and general practice. More funding targeted specifically at community care needs to be injected into the system, for example giving more funds to local authorities.

Prevention

An effective health-care system aims to provide health services to the sick and public health services to promote health and prevent the spread of disease. *Prevention* refers to actions aimed at *eradicating, eliminating* or *minimizing* the impact of disease and disability. It is often thought of in levels.

Three levels of prevention:
1. *Primary* – prevent disease.
2. *Secondary* – detect disease.
3. *Tertiary* – reduce damage.

Primary prevention

This aims to stop a disease from manifesting itself. It often calls for strategies that aim to remove or destroy agents that cause disease. Other aspects include environmental control and immunization.

Secondary prevention

This proposes to detect a disease at its earliest possible stage followed by initiating measures to cure, or prevent further progression of, the condition. The most important example in this category is screening programmes coupled with effective interventions.

Tertiary prevention

This aims to reduce the damage caused by the disease, e.g. encouraging smokers with lung cancer to quit smoking (a modifiable risk-factor that can retard progression of the disease).

Targeting a high-risk group will benefit individuals in this group, but will do little to decrease the overall burden of the disease in the population.

A population-based approach, on the other hand, which yields a smaller benefit in a larger number of individuals, may give better results. Also, there is no need to identify a high-risk group as the strategy targets all.

Health promotion

Health education is empowering individuals through increased knowledge and understanding. Unlike health promotion, there is no political advocacy. *Health promotion* interventions result in only small changes in risk factors and mortality in the general population (Fig. 6.8).

Effective health promotion relies on several factors: **P**ublic, **E**mployers, **V**oluntary groups, **A**dvertising, **M**edia, **P**rimary Care, **L**ocal authority, **I**ndustry, **G**overnment, **H**ealth services – primary/secondary and **T**raining.

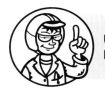

Useful mnemonic: **PE VAMP LIGHT**

The Health of the Nation

The Health of the Nation was the first national strategy for health improvement. It was adopted in 1992 and

Five approaches to health promotion

	Aim	Health promotion activity	Important values	Example: smoking
Medical	Freedom from medically defined disease and disability	Promotion of medical intervention to prevent or ameliorate ill health	Patient compliance with preventative medical procedures	*Aim*: freedom from lung disease, heart disease and other smoking-related disorders *Activity*: encourage people to seek early detection and treatment of smoking-related disorders
Behaviour change	Individual behaviour conducive to freedom from disease	Attitude and behaviour change to encourage adoption of 'healthier' lifestyle	Healthy lifestyle as defined by health promoter	*Aim*: behaviour changes from smoking to non-smoking *Activity*: persuasive education to prevent non-smokers from starting and persuade smokers to stop
Educational	Individuals with knowledge and understanding enabling well-informed decisions to be made and acted upon	Information about cause and effects of health-demoting factors Exploration of values and attitudes Development of skills required for healthy living	Individual right of free choice Health promoter's responsibility to identify educational content	*Aim*: clients will have understanding of the effect of smoking on health; they will make a decision whether or not to smoke and act on that decision *Activity*: giving information to clients about the effects of smoking; helping them to explore their own values and attitudes and come to a decision; helping them to learn how to stop smoking if they want to
Client-centred	Working with clients on the client's own terms	Working with health issues, choices and actions which clients identify Empowering the client	Client as equal Client's right to set agenda Self-empowerment of client	*Aim*: anti-smoking issues are only considered if clients identify them as a concern *Activity*: clients identify what, if anything, they want to know about it
Societal change	Physical and social environment which enables choice of healthier lifestyle	Political/social action to change physical/social environment	Right and need to make environment health-enhancing	*Aim*: make smoking socially unacceptable, so it is easier not to smoke than to smoke *Activity*: no-smoking policy in public places; cigarette sales less accessible, especially to children; promotion of non-smoking as social norm; banning tobacco advertising and sports sponsorship

Source: Ewles L & Simnet I 1995 Promoting Health: A Practical Guide. London: Scutari Press

Fig. 6.8 Five approaches to health promotion.

aims to inspire and motivate young people to change their health-related behaviours. It set out long-term objectives and measurable targets for the improvement of health in five important areas:

1. Coronary heart disease (CHD) and stroke.
2. Cancers (breast, lung, cervical and skin).
3. Mental illness.
4. HIV/AIDS and sexual health.
5. Accidents.

These areas were selected because they were major causes of premature death or avoidable ill-health and effective interventions were possible.

Saving Lives: Our Healthier Nation

This White Paper came into being in 1999. It is a comprehensive government-wide public health strategy for England. Its goals are to improve health and to reduce health inequalities. This document aims to prevent up to 300 000 untimely and unnecessary deaths by the year 2010 in the following areas:

- Cancer: reduce the death rate in people under 75 years by at least one-fifth.
- Coronary heart disease and stroke: reduce the death rate in people under 75 years by at least two-fifths.
- Accidents: reduce the death rate by at least one-fifth and serious injury by at least one-tenth.
- Mental illness: reduce the death rate from suicide and undetermined injury by at least one-fifth.

Screening

Screening is the practice of investigating apparently healthy individuals with the object of detecting unrecognized disease or its precursors in order that measures can be taken to prevent or delay the development of disease or improve prognosis.

Screening tests are generally not diagnostic. A screening test is usually cheap and simple, and aims to identify people at high risk of the condition. Further diagnostic tests are then done to confirm diagnosis.

Purpose of screening

Screening acts at all three levels of prevention:

1. Early detection of diseases where prognosis is improved by earlier treatment (for example

screening for breast cancer and offering surgical and other treatments).
2. Detection of people at increased risk of developing disease where interventions will reduce that risk (for example screening for high blood cholesterol levels and offering dietary advice and/or drug therapy).
3. Identification of people with infectious disease where treatment or other control measures will improve the outcome for the individual and prevent ongoing transmission to others (for example screening food handlers for salmonella, health workers for hepatitis B).

Mass, targeted, systematic or opportunistic

Screening can either involve the whole population (mass), or selected groups who are anticipated to have an increased prevalence of the condition (targeted). There may be a systematic programme where people are called for screening (e.g. cervical cancer) or screening may be done opportunistically when a person presents to the doctor for some other reason (e.g. blood pressure). Opportunistic screening or case-finding is advantageous in that over 90% of people will see their GP over a two-year period, so it is cost-effective whilst picking up a large proportion of cases. The problem is that there is reliance on the GP to regularly test for the condition even if the patient presents with another problem, and with current workloads, this can sometimes be forgotten (Fig. 6.9).

Criteria for screening based on WHO guidelines	
Parameter	Factor
Disease	Important health problem Well recognized pre-clinical stage Natural history understood Long period between first signs and overt disease
Diagnostic test	Valid (sensitive and specific) Simple and cheap Safe and acceptable Reliable
Diagnosis and treatment	Facilities are adequate Effective, acceptable and safe treatment available Cost effective Sustainable

Fig. 6.9 Criteria for screening based on WHO guidelines.

There are WHO guidelines for deciding when screening is appropriate, drawn up by Wilson and Jungner (1968):

1. The condition being screened for should be an important health problem.
2. The natural history should be well understood.
3. There should be a detectable early stage.
4. Treatment at an early stage should be of greater benefit than at a later stage.
5. There should be a suitable, valid test for the early stage.
6. The test should be acceptable.
7. Intervals for repeating the test should be determined.
8. There should be adequate health service provision for the extra clinical workload resulting from the screen.
9. The risks should be less than the benefits.
10. The costs should be balanced against the benefits.

The validity of a screening test is measured by its ability to do what it is supposed to do, that is distinguish between subjects with the condition and those without (Fig. 6.10).

Evaluating screening programmes

Even after a disease is determined to be appropriate for screening and a valid test becomes available, it does not necessarily follow that a widespread screening programme should be implemented. Evaluation of a potential screening programme involves consideration of three main issues outlined below.

Feasibility

Feasibility will depend on how easy it is to organize the population to attend for screening, whether the screening test is acceptable, whether facilities and resources exist to carry out the necessary diagnostic tests following screening.

Effectiveness

Effectiveness is evaluated by the extent to which implementing a screening programme affects the

Fig. 6.10 Validity of a screening test.

Validity of a screening test			
	Disease +ve	Disease −ve	
Test +ve	a	b	All Test +ve:
Test −ve	c	d	a+b
	All Disease +ve:	All Disease −ve:	All Test −ve:
	a+c	b+d	c+d

Sensitivity of screening test = proportion of true positive results detected by the screening test (%) = a/a+c

Specificity of screening test = proportion of true negative results detected by the screening test (%) = d/b+d

Positive predictive value (diagnostic value) of the test = the proportion of test positive results which are true positive results = a/a+b

Negative predictive value (diagnostic value) of the test = the proportion of test negative results which are true negative results = d/c+d

The predictive value thus indicates the likelihood of a positive or negative screening test result meaning the presence or absence of the disease respectively

Knowledge of sensitivity and specificity of a test will influence the decision whether or not to perform it

Knowledge of the predictive value will influence the view that an individual does or does not have the disease, once the test result is available

Predictive values are dependent on prevalence. Even a test with good sensitivity and specificity, when applied to a population with a low prevalence will have a low positive predictive value

subsequent outcomes. This is difficult to measure because of a number of biases that affect most of the study designs used.

Selection bias exists as people who participate in screening programmes often differ from those who do not.

Lead time bias exists because screening identifies disease that would otherwise be identified at a later stage. This may result in an apparent improvement in the length of survival due to screening which is really due to the earlier date of diagnosis.

Length bias exists as some conditions may be slower in developing to a health-threatening stage, that is, they have a longer preclinical stage. This means they are more likely to be detected at that stage, but they may also have a more favourable prognosis leading to the false conclusion that screening is beneficial in lengthening the lives of those found positive.

Screening programmes need to be tested by randomized controlled trials, partly to avoid the listed biases.

Cost

The cost of screening programmes is important. Resources for health care will always be scarce relative to competing demands. The relative cost-effectiveness of a screening programme compared with other forms of health care should, therefore, be considered. Costs relate not just to the implementation of the screening programme, but also to the further diagnostic tests and the subsequent cost of treatment. On the other hand, in the absence of screening, costs will be incurred by the treatment of patients in more advanced stages of disease (Fig. 6.11).

Ethics of screening

A screening test is a medical intervention that is done to a person who is not ill and usually to someone who has not initiated the request for the test. For this reason the ethics of carrying out screening must be carefully considered:

- The screening test can cause harm as well as providing benefits:
  - there may be a risk attached to the screening test or subsequent diagnostic test
  - a false positive result can cause unnecessary anxiety
  - there may be other unplanned effects of a positive test, e.g. the issue of diagnostic labelling that leads to the adoption of the sick role
  - a false negative result will give false reassurance.

Hence it is vital for the patient to undergo pre-test counselling.

Examples of important screening tests used today
Cervical cancer

Its objective is to detect cervical intraepithelial neoplasia. All women aged 20–64 years and whose names appear on GP lists held by health authorities are called. Screening occurs every 3–5 years. If borderline/mild dyskaryosis is seen, then the patient undergoes a re-smear. If there is moderate/severe dyskaryosis, a referral for colposcopy, laser or loop diathermy is made. Since organized screening began, the number of invasive cervical cancer cases in England and Wales has fallen by 42% in six years: from 15.4 cases per 100 000 women in 1990 to 8.9 per 100 000 by 1996, although this has not been verified by a randomized controlled trial. Also, there still seems to be a poor uptake, and the call system could be improved. Other problems include inadequately taken smears, laboratory errors and patient apathy towards recall for abnormal smears.

Breast cancer

Screening programmes aim to detect early breast cancer. The NHS Cancer Plan, published by the Department of Health in September 2000, sets out future developments in the NHS Breast Screening Programme. The programme has been extended so that women from the age of 50 years, up to and including the age of 70 years, receive routine invitations for screening. A double-view mammogram is offered at three-year intervals. Prior to 2004, the age range was 50–64 years and a single-view

Advantages and disadvantages of screening		
Screening	Opportunistic	Universal
Advantages	Cheap	Finds those who don't access health-care services regularly
Disadvantages	Identifies signs not symptoms	Stigma of recall for sexually transmitted disease
	May not access high-prevalence groups	High administration costs

Fig. 6.11 Advantages and disadvantages of screening.

119

mammogram was offered. The effects of this nationwide programme will not be available for some time. However, for all women aged 50–60 years old, there has been a reported 20% decrease in breast cancer mortality since the inception of screening, but this significant decrease has not been verified with a randomized controlled trial. The problems that need addressing include shortening the three-year interval to one year, as there appears to be a high rate of cancer in the third year. Some argue that screening needs to be increased to include those under 50 years old. There also remain issues about the safety of mammography and whether a single-view or double-view mammogram is more useful.

Other screening programmes being researched include those for prostate, ovarian and colorectal cancer.

Communicable diseases

A communicable disease is an illness caused by the *transmission* of a *specific microbial agent or its toxic products* from a *reservoir* to a susceptible *host*.

Some common terms need to be understood:
- *Occurrence* – the frequency of a disease in a population without distinguishing between the incidence and prevalence.
- *Reservoir* – the site(s) in which a disease agent normally lives and reproduces.
- *Causative agent* – a micro-organism, e.g. viruses, bacteria, whose presence is necessary for the disease to occur.
- *Transmission* – any mechanism by which an infectious agent is spread from a source or reservoir to another person. These mechanisms include:
  - *direct transmission* – via direct contact, e.g. kissing, touching, sexual intercourse. Examples of pathogens are *Staphylococcus* and *HIV*
  - *indirect transmission* – vertical transmission from mother to fetus (e.g. hepatitis B), airborne/droplet (e.g. influenza), ingestion of contaminated food/water (e.g. *Salmonella*) and vector borne (e.g. malaria).
- *Incubation period* – the time interval between exposure to the infectious agent and the appearance of the first sign or symptom of the disease.
- *Susceptibility* – the tendency of an individual to contract a disease. Affected by age, nutrition, gender, immunity and genetics.

Understanding the nature of the disease helps us to establish ways of controlling it. Generally speaking, we can use three methods to control the spread of disease:
1. *Control the agent* – involves removing agents before they enter into air, water and soil. For microbial agents, this may include prohibiting the consumption of affected foods or the use of bactericides on preparation surfaces.
2. *Control the environment* – controlling vectors, e.g. mosquito nets to prevent the spread of malaria, or treating polluted air, water and soil. Also restricting access to certain areas may help.
3. *Control the host* – protecting high-risk individuals, e.g. young, old, sick or immunosuppressed. This can be achieved by promoting personal hygiene, providing immunizations or fostering health education (Fig. 6.12).

Immunization

The aim of immunization is to provoke immunological memory to protect individuals against particular diseases. It can be defined as the protection of susceptible individuals from communicable disease by administration of a vaccine. Immunization can be *passive* (short-term, e.g. immunoglobulins or antibodies) or *active* (acquired naturally after recovery from infection with the causal organism or induced artificially via a vaccine).

A vaccine is an immunobiological agent injected into the body to stimulate an immune response. There are four types:
1. *Inactivated/killed vaccines* – made from whole organisms killed during manufacture, e.g. pertussis.
2. *Live vaccines* – made from living organisms, which are either the disease-causing organisms whose virulence has been reduced by attenuation, e.g. MMR, or less virulent organisms of a species antigenically related to the causal agent, e.g. BCG.
3. *Toxoids* – produced from artificially created, but harmless bacterial toxins, e.g. tetanus.
4. *Component/sub-unit vaccines* – contain a component antigen(s) of the target organism required to evoke a suitable immune response, e.g. influenza.

Live vaccines are given in a single dose and have a longer duration of immunity. However, they may be

Primary tuberculosis as an example of communicable disease control	
Communicable disease parameter	Primary tuberculosis
Occurrence	5700 cases/year
Reservoir	Primarily human
Transmission	Mainly droplet nuclei
Incubation period	Often asymptomatic; casual short-term exposure is less likely to transmit the disease
Susceptibility – risk factors	Poor nutrition Poor living conditions Some sections of society, e.g. alcoholics, undernourished, some ethnic minority communities, the elderly, and HIV positive individuals Farm workers who drink unpasteurized milk Gastrectomy patients
Control	Identifying and treating those who already have the disease, to shorten their infection and to stop it being passed on to other people BCG vaccine

less stable and revert to the virulent strain and cause disease in the immunosuppressed.

Inactivated vaccines are given in multiple doses and need a booster. They confer shorter immunity and are stable.

Herd immunity is the immunity of a group or community. For example, if enough children acquire immunity to measles, owing to vaccination, the measles virus loses the ability to circulate in the community (Fig. 6.13).

Some of the factors associated with poor vaccine uptake are:
- Socio-demographic variables.
- Deprived, inner-city living.
- Mobile families.
- Birth order, large families.
- Children with chronic illnesses.
- Ethnicity.
- Personal variables.
- Attitudes of parents.
- Attitudes of professionals.
- Health service variables – generally good in the UK, but be aware of some limitations.
- Poor coordination (private and public sectors).
- Unclear responses, e.g. questioning the potential harms of the MMR vaccine.
- Access to guidelines and policies.

In the UK, it is a legal requirement for health authorities to be informed of certain 'notifiable diseases'. The Consultant in Communicable Disease Control (CCDC) is responsible for prevention, control and surveillance of communicable diseases. The Public Health Laboratory Service (PHLS) provides support to these doctors at a national level (Figs 6.14, 6.15).

Expanded programme of immunization (EPI) – European (UK) schedule	
2, 3 and 4 months old	Diphtheria/tetanus/polio (DTP) Polio *Haemophilus influenzae* type b (Hib)
12–15 months	Meningitis C vaccine (conjugated) Measles/mumps/rubella (MMR)
3–5 years (pre-school)	DTP Polio MMR
11–13 years	BCG
12–15 years	MMR
15 years old	Diphtheria/tetanus (D/T) Polio

Also: BCG at birth in at-risk population; hepatitis B at 0, 1, 2, and 12 months old if born to a carrier mother.

Fig. 6.13 Expanded programme of immunization (EPI) – European (UK) schedule.

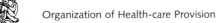

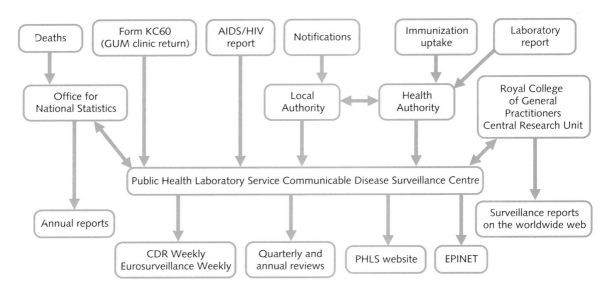

Fig. 6.14 Flow of information about communicable diseases in England and Wales.
Source: Donaldson LJ, Donaldson RJ 2000 Essential Public Health. Berkshire: Petroc Press, p. 358

Management of disease outbreaks

The impact of disease can be described as follows:
- *Outbreak* – an epidemic restricted to a localized increase in the incidence of disease, e.g. in a county.
- *Epidemic* – an increase in the incidence of a disease above that which is ever-present in a population.
- *Endemic* – the incidence of a disease that is continuously present in a population.
- *Pandemic* – an epidemic occurring across international boundaries and affecting a large number of people.

Surveillance is 'the continued watchfulness over the distribution and trends in the incidence of disease through the systematic collection, consolidation and evaluation of morbidity and mortality reports and other relevant data' (Langmuir 1963).

Sources of surveillance data include:
- Statutory notifications.
- Laboratory reports.
- Royal College of General Practitioners sentinel reporting system.
- Hospital Episode Statistics (HES) data.
- Death certificates.
- Vaccine use.
- Sickness absence.

- Special systems: clinical HIV reporting, which is voluntary to the Communicable Disease Surveillance Centre (CDSC), the British

Notifiable diseases

Acute encephalitis	Ophthalmia neonatorum
Acute poliomyelitis	Paratyphoid fever
Anthrax	Plague
Cholera	Rabies
Diphtheria	Relapsing fever
Dysentery (amoebic or bacillary)	Rubella
Food poisoning	Scarlet fever
HIV	Tetanus
Leprosy	Tuberculosis
Leptospirosis	Typhoid fever
Malaria	Typhus
Measles	Viral haemorrhagic fever
Meningococcal septicaemia (without meningitis)	Whooping cough
Mumps	Yellow fever

Fig. 6.15 Notifiable diseases.

Paediatrics Surveillance Unit and the Creutzfeldt-Jakob Disease (CJD) Surveillance Unit (important as cases rise).

Principles of surveillance
- Systematic collection of data.
- Analyses of data to produce statistics.
- Interpretation of statistics.
- Distribution of this information to those who require it for action. Feedback is via Communicable Disease Report (CDR) Weekly, information services, internet information sites, e.g. Public Health Laboratory Service (PHLS).
- Continuing surveillance to evaluate action.

The CDSC publishes reports of notifications of diseases.

Steps in controlling an outbreak
1. Preliminary assessment in outbreak investigation – to confirm the existence of an outbreak. Consult the CDSC. If further investigations are needed, review the literature and survey the data. Form an outbreak control team. Also generate the initial hypothesis and initiate immediate control measures as necessary, for example stop symptomatic food handlers from working.
2. Case definition and identification – define 'cases' in terms of time/place/person/symptoms/laboratory results and define the population at risk.
3. Descriptive study – collect and analyse data. Draw the epidemic curve and generate the hypothesis. The aim is to link the cases to a source.
4. Analytical study – can be done using a *cohort study* (population is known, e.g. guests at party) or a *case-control study* for a large population. The aims are to test the generated hypothesis and to attempt to overcome bias.
5. Verify hypothesis – by using food and environmental samples sent to the microbiology lab.
6. Institute control measures:
   a. Remove source – close outlet, isolate and treat cases, destroy/treat food
   b. Protect persons at risk – improve hygiene and prophylaxis
   c. Prevent recurrence – recommendations and guidelines.
7. Communicate – during the investigation give updated information to the public and professionals. Upon conclusion, publish a report for those involved and interested individuals.

Some of the steps above may be carried out simultaneously, so keep a record of the date and time.

- Describe the evolution of the NHS since its birth in 1948, including the major reforms undertaken.
- Briefly discuss the organization of the NHS.
- Outline the strengths and weaknesses of the NHS system in the 21st century.
- Compare the different systems for organizing health-care delivery.
- Discuss the process of clinical governance.
- Show how the boundaries between medical, nursing and other health-care professions have changed since the early 20th century.
- Outline the different types of prevention.
- Outline the importance of care in the community.
- Describe the initiatives instituted by the government to promote the general health of the population.
- Evaluate screening as a tool to detect unrecognized disease or improve prognosis.
- Discuss the important screening tests used in the UK and any impact they have had on the pattern of the disease.
- Briefly discuss the different methods of controlling the spread of disease.
- Outline the different factors that can affect the uptake of a vaccine.
- Explain how you would manage the outbreak of a disease.
- Briefly discuss the role of surveillance for communicable diseases.

References

Carr-Saunders AM, Wilson PA 1933 The Professions. Oxford: Clarendon Press

Field M 1973 The concept of the 'health system' at the macrosociological level. Sociology, science and medicine 7: 763–85

Fitzpatrick R 2003 Organizing and funding health care. In: Scambler G (ed.) Sociology as Applied to Medicine, 5th edn. Edinburgh: Saunders, pp. 292–307

Langmuir AD 1963 The surveillance of communicable diseases of national importance. New England Journal of Medicine 268: 182–92

Larson MS 1977 The Rise of Professionalism: A Sociological Analysis. Berkeley, CA: University of California Press

MacDonald KM 1995 The Sociology of Professions. London: Sage

Wilson JMG, Jungner G 1968 Principles and Practice of Screening for Disease. Geneva: World Health Organization

Further reading

Farmer R, Lawrenson R, Miller D 2001 Lecture Notes on Epidemiology and Public Health Medicine, 4th edn. Oxford: Blackwell Science

Jones IR 2003 Health professions. In: Scambler G (ed.) Sociology as Applied to Medicine, 5th edn. Edinburgh: Saunders, pp. 235–47

Mays N 2003 Origins and development of the National Health Service. In: Scambler G (ed.) Sociology as Applied to Medicine, 5th edn. Edinburgh: Saunders, pp. 205–34

Vetters N, Matthews I 1999 Components of health care – preventative health care, health promotion and screening. In: Vetters N, Matthews I (eds) Epidemiology and Public Health Medicine. Edinburgh: Churchill Livingstone, pp. 215–20

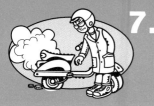

This chapter considers inequalities by social class, gender, ethnicity and age.

Impact of social class

There is a long tradition in Britain of analysing national statistics to shed light on the nature and causes of social inequalities in health. This goes back at least to William Farr in 1837, when the General Register Office was set up. Farr, as the first Superintendent of Statistics, clearly believed that it was the responsibility of the national office not just to record deaths, but to uncover underlying linkages which might help to prevent disease and suffering in the future.

In the 19th century the associations between various occupations and health were put down to:
- Specific work-related hazards.
- Variation of income – which affected the provision of nutrition and housing.

In 1942 the Beveridge Report set out a national programme of policies to combat the 'five giants of Want, Disease, Ignorance, Squalor and Idleness'. In 1977 the Research Working Group on Inequalities in Health, chaired by Sir Douglas Black, was set up. The resulting 'Black Report' presented in 1980 attempted to explain trends in inequalities in health. It argued that inequalities in health were a result of inequalities in society. While the recommendations of this report had a significant effect in academic circles, it arguably failed to produce change in political policies (health inequalities grew through the Thatcher years).

In 1997, the new Labour government set up an independent inquiry chaired by Sir Donald Acheson. The Acheson Inquiry, published in 1998, identified the following as areas where policy could redress health inequalities by tackling socioeconomic factors (see also p. 127):
1. Poverty, income, tax and benefits.
2. Education.
3. Employment.
4. Housing and environment.
5. Mobility, transport and pollution.
6. Nutrition.

Health inequality
- Life expectancy at birth for a boy is about five years less in the two lowest social classes than in the two highest, at 70 and 75 years respectively.
- Each of the main disease groups shows a wide health gap among men, with those in the highest two social classes experiencing lower mortality than men in the lowest two.
- Men aged between 20 and 64 years from the bottom social class are three times more likely to die from coronary heart disease and stroke than those in the top social class.
- Mortality from all major causes has been found to be consistently higher than average among unemployed men; unemployed women have higher mortality from coronary heart disease and suicide.
- Children from manual households are more likely to suffer from chronic sickness than children from non-manual households. Similarly for tooth decay.
- Men in manual classes are about 40% more likely to report a long-standing illness that limits their activities than those in non-manual classes.

The recommendations made by the Report insist on input from many government departments – not just the Department of Health – in order to reduce health inequalities.

In 1999, the government outlined its strategy for addressing health inequalities in the document *Saving Lives: Our Healthier Nation*. It claimed its aims were to:

The Acheson Inquiry, which published its Report in November 1998, confirmed that for many aspects of health, inequality has generally worsened in the last few decades, especially in the 1980s and early 1990s.

- Improve the health of **everyone.**
- Improve the health of the **worst off** in particular.

They set the targets to tackle four major areas of health by 2010. These were:
- Cancer: to reduce the death rate in people under 75 by at least one-fifth.
- Coronary heart disease and stroke: to reduce the death rate in people under 75 by at least two-fifths.
- Accidents: to reduce the death rate by at least one-fifth and serious injury by at least one-tenth.
- Mental illness: to reduce the death rate from suicide and undetermined injury by at least one-fifth.

Social stratification

Social stratification refers to the way in which an individual who is disadvantaged in one area of life tends to be disadvantaged in others as well. Thus an individual with a low income probably also has a reduced access to quality housing, education and health-care services. The concept of 'social class' has been used to describe social stratification within British society. The stratification most widely used in the general population is that of Scambler & Blane (2003, p. 111):
- 'Working-class' – characterized by earning weekly wages in manual jobs; renting homes, mainly from a local authority; and the aspiration of getting their children in a good job as soon as they are allowed to leave school.
- 'Middle-class' – characterized by earning monthly salaries in non-manual jobs; borrowing money to buy their own homes; and encouraging their children to gain as much formal education as possible.

Most medical research uses a scale with a greater number of categories – the Registrar General's classification. This divides the population into five social classes based on occupation according to skill level and general social standing (Fig. 7.1).

Registrar General's classification of social classes

Social class	Description	Examples
I	Professional	Accountant
		Doctor
		Lawyer
II	Intermediate	Manager
		School teacher
		Nurse
IIIN	Skilled non-manual	Clerical worker
		Secretary
		Shop Assistant
IIIM	Skilled manual	Bus driver
		Coal-face worker
		Carpenter
IV	Semi-skilled manual	Agricultural worker
		Bus conductor
		Postman
V	Unskilled manual	Labourer
		Cleaner
		Dock worker

Fig. 7.1 Registrar General's classification of social classes.

Within this classification:
- Men are allocated a social class according to their occupation.
- Married women according to their husband's occupation.
- Single women according to their own occupation.
- Children according to that of their father.
- The unemployed/retired according to that of the last significant period of employment.

Criticisms of the Registrar General's classification include (Scambler & Blane 2003, p. 112):
1. The classification is a measure of social status rather than income.
2. Each class is not internally homogeneous – for example, 'manager' in social class II includes the owner of a corner-shop and the managing directors of multinational companies.
3. The classification is inadequate in the way it deals with women. A married woman is classified

according to the class of her husband, even though her income may be decisive in determining the standard of living of the family.

4. The relevancy of the classification has been questioned given the flexible nature of labour markets, job insecurity and unemployment rates.

Variations in health according to social class

Even though overall death rates have fallen considerably over the past 200 years, the difference between 'rich' and 'poor' has persisted. The Acheson Inquiry observed:

> Inequalities in health exist, whether measured in terms of mortality, life expectancy or health status; whether categorised by socioeconomic measures or by ethnic group or gender. Recent efforts to compare the level and nature of health inequalities in international terms indicate that Britain is generally around the middle of comparable western countries, depending on the socioeconomic and inequality indicators used.

The Acheson Inquiry also reported the following:
- Over the last 20 years, death rates have fallen among both men and women and across all social groups.
- The difference in rates between those at the top and bottom of the social scale has widened.
- In the early 1970s, the mortality rate among men of working age was almost twice as high for those in class V (unskilled) as for those in class I (professional). By the early 1990s, it was almost three times higher (Fig. 7.2). This increasing differential is because, although rates fell overall, they fell more among the high social classes than the low social classes. Between the early 1970s and the early 1990s, rates fell by about 40% for classes I and II, about 30% for classes IIIN, IIIM and IV, but by only 10% for class V. So not only did the differential between the top and the bottom increase, but the increase happened across the whole spectrum of social classes.
- Both class I and class V cover only a small proportion of the population, at the extremes of the social scale. Combining class I with class II and class IV with class V allows comparisons of larger sections of the population. Among both men and women aged 35–64 years, overall death rates fell for each group between 1976–81 and 1986–92 (Fig. 7.3). At the same time, the gap between classes I and II and classes IV and V increased. In the late 1970s, death rates were 53% higher among men in classes IV and V compared with those in classes I and II. In the late 1980s, they were 68% higher. Among women, the differential increased from 50% to 55%.
- These growing differences across the social spectrum were apparent for many of the major causes of death, including coronary heart disease, stroke, lung cancer and suicides among men, and respiratory disease and lung cancer among women.
- Death rates can be summarized into average life expectancy at birth. For men in classes I and II combined, life expectancy increased by two years between the late 1970s and the late 1980s. For those in classes IV and V combined, the increase was smaller, 1.4 years. The difference between those at the top and bottom of the social class scale in the late 1980s was five years, 75 years compared with 70 years. For women, the differential was smaller, 80 years compared with 77 years. Improvements in life expectancy have been greater, over the period from the late 1970s to the late 1980s, for women in classes I and II than for those in classes IV and V: two years compared to one year.
- A good measure of inequality among older people is life expectancy at age 65 years. Again, in the late 1980s, this was considerably higher among those in higher social classes, and the differential increased over the period from the late 1970s to the late 1980s, particularly for women.

With regards to morbidity, the Acheson Inquiry stated:
- There is little evidence that the population is experiencing less morbidity or disability than 10 or 20 years ago. There has been a slight increase in self-reported long-standing illness and limiting long-standing illness, and socioeconomic differences are substantial.
- Among men, major accidents are more common in the manual classes for those aged under 55 years. Between 55 and 64 years, the non-manual classes have higher major accident rates. For women, there are no differences in accident rates until after the age of 75 years, when those women in the non-manual group have higher rates of major accidents.
- Ten per cent of men in classes IV and V were dependent on alcohol compared to 5% in classes I and II.

In addition, the 1997 Health Inequalities Decennial supplement showed that:

- There is a social class gradient in the prevalence of hypertension (Fig. 7.4).
- GP consultations are higher among manual than non-manual classes.
- In both sexes, members of social class I had more positive health-related behaviours – such as not smoking, regular dental and ophthalmic check-ups, a balanced diet, and regular exercise – than social class V.

Why do such profound differences in health exist?

The Black Report proposed four explanations as to why there was an association between social class and health. These were:

1. *Artefact*: that is, the association is spurious because of the way the concepts involved are measured:

   a. One example of this is numerator-denominator bias: this comes about because mortality rates (in the Black Report) relied on

Fig. 7.2 European standardized mortality rates by social class, selected causes, men aged 20–64, England and Wales, selected years.

European standardized mortality rates by social class, selected causes, men aged 20–64, England and Wales, selected years

All causes (rates per 100 000)				Lung cancer (rates per 100 000)			
Social class	Year			Social class	Year		
	1970–71	1979–83	1991–93		1970–71	1979–83	1991–93
I - Professional	500	373	280	I - Professional	41	26	17
II - Managerial	526	425	300	II - Managerial	52	39	24
III(N) - Skilled (non-manual)	637	522	426	III(N) - Skilled (non-manual)	63	46	34
III(M) - Skilled (manual)	683	580	493	III(M) - Skilled (manual)	90	72	54
IV - Partly skilled	721	639	492	IV - Partly skilled	93	76	52
V - Unskilled	897	910	806	V - Unskilled	109	108	82
England and Wales	624	549	419	England and Wales	73	60	39

Coronary heart disease (rates per 100 000)				Stroke (rates per 100 000)			
Social class	Year			Social class	Year		
	1970–71	1979–83	1991–93		1970–71	1979–83	1991–93
I - Professional	195	144	81	I - Professional	35	20	14
II - Managerial	197	168	92	II - Managerial	37	23	13
III(N) - Skilled (non-manual)	245	208	136	III(N) - Skilled (non-manual)	41	28	19
III(M) - Skilled (manual)	232	218	159	III(M) - Skilled (manual)	45	34	24
IV - Partly skilled	232	227	156	IV - Partly skilled	46	37	25
V - Unskilled	243	287	235	V - Unskilled	59	55	45
England and Wales	209	201	127	England and Wales	40	30	20

Fig. 7.2 (*Continued*)

European standardized mortality rates by social class, selected causes, men aged 20–64, England and Wales, selected years

Accidents, poisonings, violence (rates per 100 000)				Suicide and undetermined injury (rates per 100 000)			
Social class	Year			Social class	Year		
	1970–71	1979–83	1991–93		1970–71	1979–83	1991–93
I - Professional	23	17	13	I - Professional	16	16	13
II - Managerial	25	20	13	II - Managerial	13	15	14
III(N) - Skilled (non-manual)	25	21	17	III(N) - Skilled (non-manual)	17	18	20
III(M) - Skilled (manual)	34	27	24	III(M) - Skilled (manual)	12	16	21
IV - Partly skilled	39	35	24	IV - Partly skilled	18	23	23
V - Unskilled	67	63	52	V - Unskilled	32	44	47
England and Wales	34	28	22	England and Wales	15	20	22

Source: An Independent Inquiry into Inequalities in Health Report, London, HMSO
http://www.archive.official-documents.co.uk/document/doh/ih/tab3.htm

figures from two different sources. The number of deaths in each social class came from death registration. The number of individuals in each class came from census data. Any attempt to 'promote' oneself in the census would lead to artificially increased rates in social classes IV and V.

But:

- A longitudinal study of 1% of the 1971 census population showed this is unlikely.

b. Infant mortality and social class: there is a question as to whether the association with infant mortality is derived in a circular fashion. When originally conceived, a number of factors were used to assign each occupation to a social class, which included housing behaviour, education and wealth – factors that are known to have an influence on infant mortality. So those factors that cause infant mortality are used to determine a low social class status. To then claim that low social class status causes increased infant mortality is artefactual.

But:

- Social class grading depends on a number of factors – so it isn't entirely arbitrary in this manner.

2. *Social selection*: this explanation argues that rather than social class determining health, health determines social class. The proposed mechanism for this is that if people fall ill, they are unable to secure employment in classes I and II. For example, a schizophrenic with active disease may not be able to work as a doctor or lawyer, but could probably find some semi- or unskilled work. It seems probable that the healthy are socially mobile upwardly, and the unhealthy move downwards.

But:

- Is this mechanism sufficiently powerful to explain the whole social class gradient? Probably not because (Scambler & Blane 2003, p. 118):
  - the gradient is already present in children – prior to social mobility
  - the gradients are present after social mobility – in retirement
  - the class differences are roughly the same for acute and chronic diseases – if they were due to social mobility, it would be expected that they would be greater in chronic diseases where there is more time to move downwards
  - social mobility tends to occur before serious diseases become prevalent

Fig. 7.3 Age-standardized mortality rates per 100 000 by social class, selected causes, men and women aged 35–64, England and Wales, 1976–92.

Age-standardized mortality rates per 100 000 by social class, selected causes, men and women aged 35–64, England and Wales, 1976–92

	Women (35–64)			Men (35–64)		
	1976–81	1981–85	1986–92	1976–81	1981–85	1986–92
All causes						
I/II	338	344	270	621	539	455
IIIN	371	387	305	860	658	484
IIIM	467	396	356	802	691	624
IV/V	508	445	418	951	824	764
Ratio IV/V:I/II	1.5	1.29	1.55	1.53	1.53	1.68
Coronary heart disease						
I/II	39	45	29	246	185	160
IIIN	56	57	39	382	267	162
IIIM	85	67	59	309	269	231
IV/V	105	76	78	363	293	266
Ratio IV/V:I/II	2.69	1.69	2.69	1.48	1.58	1.66
Breast cancer						
I/II	52	74	52			
IIIN	75	71	49			
IIIM	61	57	46			
IV/V	47	50	54			
Ratio IV/V:I/II	0.90	0.68	1.04			

Source: Independent Inquiry into Inequalities in Health Report 1997 London: TSO. http://www.archive.official-documents.co.uk/document/doh/ih/tab3.htm

Fig. 7.4 Table showing variation in morbidity between social classes.

Table showing variation in morbidity between social classes

Condition	Men		Women	
	I	V	I	V
Long-standing illness	31% (in 45–64 year olds)	53% (in 45–64 year olds)	36% (in 45–64 year olds)	50% (in 45–64 year olds)
Obesity (BMI>30)	10%	13%	12%	21%
Hypertension	16%	24%	22%	26%
Neurotic disorders	–	–	15% (social class I & II)	24% (social class IV & V)

– incapacity does not always lead to downward mobility – it may lead to early retirement, unemployment or moving to less-demanding jobs – these may involve a reduction in income but not a reclassification on the Registrar General's classification.

3. *Behavioural/cultural*: It is possible to consider the middle and working classes as having different cultures. As Armstrong (1989) points out: 'they have different habits, read different newspapers, watch different television programmes, have different leisure activities, have different outlooks on life, and so on'. Health-related behaviours include:

a. Smoking:
   i. In 1974, 50% of men and 40% of women smoked cigarettes
   ii. In 1996 less than 30% of men and women smoke – this breaks down into:
   men: 12 % (social class I) and 41% (social class V)
   women: 11 % (social class I) and 36% (social class V)

b. Alcohol:
   i. The proportion of women who drank more than 14 units of alcohol a week rose from 9% in 1984 to 14% in 1996
   ii. In spite of the major class differences in dependence on alcohol in men, there are very small differences in the reported quantities consumed. This is not the case among women where higher consumption is related to higher social class.

c. Physical exercise:
   i. Women: no differences in levels of physical activity across the social classes.
   ii. Men: higher proportions in the manual classes have a high level of physical activity than in the non-manual classes. However, some of this difference is due to work-related physical activity. Men in non-manual occupations have higher rates of leisure-time physical activity.

d. Diet:
   i. People in lower socioeconomic groups tend to eat less fruit and vegetables, and less food that is rich in dietary fibre.
   ii. One aspect of dietary behaviour that affects the health of infants is the incidence of breast feeding. Six weeks after birth, almost three-quarters of babies in class I households are still breast-fed. This declines with class to less than one-quarter of babies in class V. The differences between classes in rates of breast-feeding at six weeks has narrowed slightly between 1985 and 1995.

The implications of cultural explanations for health inequalities are twofold:

- They may not be eradicated by a reduction in economic inequalities alone.
- Perhaps they *should* not be eradicated – as Armstrong points out: 'If . . . a working class man smokes because he finds pleasure in the activity, and he is less concerned about the long-term consequences, do middle class health professionals have a right to tell him that his values are mistaken and that he should substitute deferred gratification for immediate? There is evidence that cigarette smoking is an integral component of the lifestyle of many working class people; is it morally right to try and change this for a middle class value?'

4. *Materialist*: this explanation is the one favoured by the Black Report as being of the greatest significance. The Acheson Inquiry also subscribed to this sort of explanation, barely mentioning artefact and social selection. It maintained that the association between social class and health is caused by the associated levels of material deprivation. Examples of this include:

a. Lack of material possessions – including clothes and food
b. Poor housing – damp, overcrowding and hypothermia (especially for older people) contribute to poor health. Housing may be situated in areas with high levels of atmospheric or environmental pollution and there may not be suitable areas for children to play outside
c. Poor access – to education and health care. Housing prices tend to be increased in areas where good schools are based – less-well-achieving schools are located in areas of poor housing. The children of poor families are less able to use education as a route out of the cycle of poverty. Tudor Hart (1971) introduced the concept of the 'Inverse Care Law' claiming health care was least available where it was most needed (i.e. by the working class) and, therefore, it was under-utilized by the lower social classes. This is somewhat supported by data showing that the lower social classes are less likely to use screening, dental care, postnatal examinations and so on.

Further study has extended the explanatory power of the materialist perspective. It has been demonstrated that physical and social disadvantage accumulates over the course of a lifetime to produce accrued ill effects:

- Low parental social class is associated with health disadvantages in utero, and in the early years of life – for example, poor nutrition, increased incidence of chronic illness in childhood, failure to thrive and slow growth leading to short stature for age and sex.

- Social factors – such as family conflict, poor housing and overcrowding – can also lead to poor health outcomes. Children from such families fare less well at school – poor educational achievement results in poor job prospects and an increased likelihood of long-term unemployment. Thus, childhood disadvantage readily leads to poor socio-economic status and disadvantage in adulthood.
- Low educational achievement is also associated with early parenthood, and lone parenthood (mostly lone mothers), which in turn is associated with increased poverty. In turn the new generation of children born are exposed to significant disadvantage. It has been found that whilst in the 1970s 10% of children lived in poverty, by the late 1990s the proportion was 35%.
- Government policy, particularly in respect to taxation and social security benefits, has played a significant role in this increase. State benefits have declined in relative value to the incomes of those higher up the income ladder.
- Relative deprivation (rather than absolute deprivation) has been increasing in the UK. That is, the gap between the rich and the poor has been getting larger.

An important concept is the 'cycle of poverty'. In Victorian days 'poverty caused disease which caused poverty'. With the welfare state this is probably less of a problem now; however, being disadvantaged in one area of life is associated with being disadvantaged in others.

Relative vs. absolute deprivation

Marmot (2003) discusses the importance of social gradients within societies leading to ill health. He argues there are three ways in which socioeconomic position could be linked to health (Fig. 7.5):

1. Money.
2. Status.
3. Power.

He argues that whilst a high income is associated with good health, it is merely an indicator for position within society (status) – which is the most important predictor of health. He draws a comparison between men in Costa Rica (average income $2000 per annum and life expectancy of 74 years) and black American men (average income $26 000 per annum and life expectancy of 66 years). Even adjusting for the fact that more can be bought for less in Costa Rica than in the USA (such that the $2000 is probably equivalent to around $6600 in the USA), US black men still have a lower life expectancy even though they have an income that is almost four times greater. Marmot argues that this is due to the relatively low status occupied by black American men within US society rather than due to absolute poverty. The mechanism by which this may occur is the relative disadvantage in terms of income within a society. Marmot suggests that this 'relative inequality . . . may correspond to absolute discrimination and social exclusion'.

Marmot goes on to describe how health differences occur along a social gradient even amongst a single socioeconomic group. In his studies of civil servants (the Whitehall studies), he has displayed an increased mortality and morbidity with progressive loss of control over their jobs or loss of power.

Reducing inequality between social classes I and V

As mentioned above, the Acheson Inquiry mentioned six key areas where policy improvements could help to reduce the health inequalities in this country. The government addressed these areas in their paper *Saving Lives: Our Healthier Nation*, as follows:

1. Poverty, income, tax and benefits:
   a. introduction of the minimum wage
   b. increased benefits for single mothers and older people
   c. a new system of tax credits for parents.
2. Education:
   a. the *Healthy Schools* programme, which involves partnerships between local health and education authorities to provide 'healthy' school environments and information for children about health.
   b. educational resources, such as a health website for children, have been set up (www.wiredforhealth.gov.uk)
   c. *cooking for kids* – an in-school educational programme which teaches the basics of healthy eating and cooking.

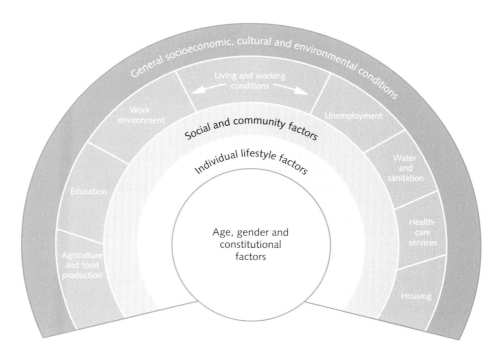

Fig. 7.5 The main determinants of health.
Source: Independent Inquiry into Inequalities in Health Report. London: TSO. http://www.archive.official-documents.co.uk/document/doh/ih/tab2.htm

3. Employment:
   a. the *New Deal* – to encourage people off welfare and into the workforce
   b. *The Healthy Workplace Initiative* (1999) to encourage healthy practices in the workplace.
4. Housing and environment:
   a. benefits for fuel
   b. benefits for making houses energy efficient
   c. the *New Deal for Communities* – money given to improve neighbourhoods – to develop social cohesion and strong social networks.
5. Mobility, transport and pollution:
   a. encouraging local authorities to prioritize transport issues in disadvantaged areas
   b. encourage local service providers, e.g. GP practices, pharmacists, to establish services in disadvantaged areas.

6. Nutrition:
   a. improve access to affordable healthy foods for people on low incomes
   b. restrict advertising of food high in salt, fat and sugar targeted at children
   c. 'five-a-day' advertising campaign to increase the amount of fruit and vegetables people eat
   d. reduce salt and fat content in processed foods.

Many of these policies are 'upstream' policies designed to have a wide range of consequences – including benefits to health. The Acheson Inquiry recommended both 'upstream' and 'downstream' policies – those that deal with wider influences on health inequalities such as income distribution, education, public safety, housing, work environment, employment, social networks, transport and pollution, as well as those which have narrower impacts, such as on healthy behaviours.

Health inequalities and social class
- The materialist perspective sees health inequalities as being due to inequalities in wealth.
- Inequalities in health are associated with many social and environmental factors.
- The Acheson Inquiry did not consider artefact and self selection to be significant causes of inequalities in health between social classes – research in the 1980s and 1990s showed that materialist and behavioural explanations were significant in causing health inequalities.
- Social inequality leads to a life-time accumulation of disadvantages that contribute to poor health outcomes. On this the Department of Health has concluded:

  It is likely that cumulative differential exposure to health damaging or health promoting physical and social environments is the main explanation for the observed variations in health and life expectancy.

Definitions of sex and gender
- Sex: refers to the classes of 'male' and 'female' as determined by biology.
- Gender: refers to the classes of 'masculine' and 'feminine' as socially and culturally constructed.

of the two sexes, rather it is due to the combined effects of biological, social and cultural influences.

Levels of inequality
Mortality

It has often been said that 'women get sick and men die'. In general this is true; however, it belies a rather more complex picture of the gender biases in mortality and morbidity (Fig. 7.6). Mortality is the easier of the two to measure – death being a far more objective measure. Men die younger and in greater numbers in all age groups:

- Life expectancy for males: 74.3 years (EU average 74.3)
- Life expectancy for females: 79.5 years (EU average 80.7).

In childhood the mortality in males is raised due to accidental deaths – especially due to poisoning and injury due to causes such as drowning, road-traffic accidents and fire (Fig. 7.7). The difference between male and female deaths rises to a maximum in the 20–24-year-old group, where male mortality is 2.8 times that of female. The major causes of this disparity are road-traffic accidents, other accidents and suicide (Fig. 7.8). Figure 7.9 outlines the different causes of death in men and women.

Gender differences

Like social class, gender affects one's long-term health. This is not simply due to the different biological aspects

Fig. 7.6 Standardized mortality rates, by gender, all ages, England and Wales, 1971–96.
Source: Independent Inquiry into Inequalities in Health Report. London: TSO. http//www. archive.official-documents.co.uk/document/doh/ih/fig10.htm

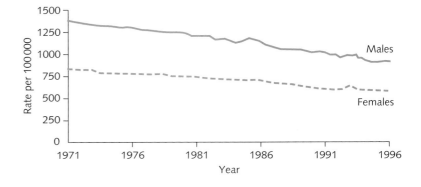

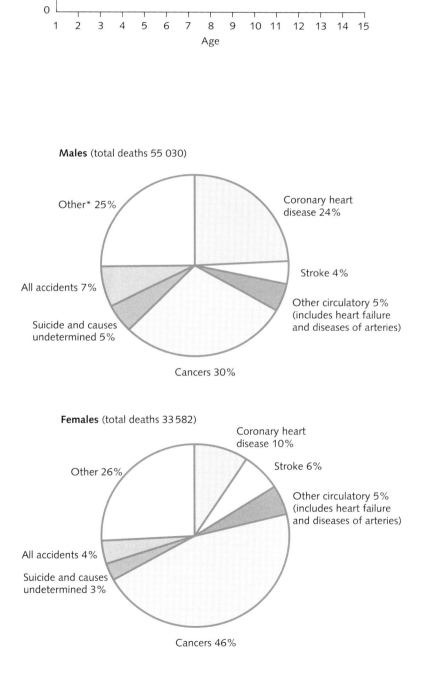

Fig. 7.7 Age-specific mortality rates, children, England and Wales, 1991–95.
Source: Independent Inquiry into Inequalities in Health Report. London: TSO. http://www.archive.official-documents.co.uk/document/doh/ih/fig11.htm

Males (total deaths 55 030)

Other* 25%

Coronary heart disease 24%

Stroke 4%

Other circulatory 5% (includes heart failure and diseases of arteries)

All accidents 7%

Suicide and causes undetermined 5%

Cancers 30%

Fig. 7.8 Major causes of mortality under 65 years by sex, England 1996.
Source: Independent Inquiry into Inequalities in Health Report. London: TSO. http://www.archive.official-documents.co.uk/document/doh/ohnation/fig15.htm
*Deaths occurring at ages under 28 days are included in the totals but are not allocated to a specific cause of death. These are therefore included in 'Other'. The major categories presented in this figure are those which have been identified as priority areas for *Our Healthier Nation*. All remaining causes of death have been assigned to the 'Other' category.

Females (total deaths 33 582)

Coronary heart disease 10%

Stroke 6%

Other circulatory 5% (includes heart failure and diseases of arteries)

Other 26%

All accidents 4%

Suicide and causes undetermined 3%

Cancers 46%

Causes of death in men and women			
Disease category – male (per 100 000 population)	Death rate	Disease category – female (per 100 000 population)	Death rate
Ischaemic heart disease	227.8	Ischaemic heart disease	175.0
Cerebrovascular disease	88.9	Cerebrovascular disease	134.9
Lung cancer	69.2	Pneumonia	72.4
Bronchitis	51.3	Breast cancer	43.0
Pneumonia	49.4	Lung cancer	41.4
Prostate cancer	34.7	Bronchitis	38.9
Bowel cancer	29.1	Bowel cancer	24.7
All accidents	23.9	All accidents	17.6
Stomach cancer	13.5	Diabetes mellitus	11.8
Chronic liver disease and cirrhosis	12.7	Pancreatic cancer	11.7v
Diabetes mellitus	11.4	Chronic liver disease and cirrhosis	7.2
Pancreatic cancer	11.3	Stomach cancer	7.0
Suicide	10.1	Uterine cancer	3.7
		Suicide	2.8

Fig. 7.9 Causes of death in men and women.

In general the gender differences are greatest in areas of relative deprivation, and least in affluent areas. However, remarkably, affluent men still have a greater risk of mortality than deprived women.

Morbidity

Morbidity highlights an apparent paradox: that males have higher mortality rates, but females have higher rates of morbidity. However, the broad assumption that females experience more ill health than males conceals specific gender differences in both directions.

Childhood and adolescence

- Boys are more likely to report long-standing illness (18% M:15% F).
- Boys are 30–40% more likely than girls to have consulted at a general practice for serious conditions, but about 10% less likely to have done so for minor conditions.
- While boys have higher rates of chronic physical illness in childhood, this pattern is reversed in early to mid-adolescence, when there are higher rates for girls.

Female longevity
Female longevity has not always been manifest:
- It is thought that there was a substantial male advantage in longevity in the 16th and 17th centuries.
- In the first half of the 19th century male and female life expectancies were more or less equal.
- By the 1960s women were living about six years longer than men.
- The gap in life expectancy may be closing once again.
- The major change in female mortality is due to changing patterns of child-bearing and the reduction in maternal mortality.
- The levels of female mortality in the developing world resemble 19th-century mortality rates in the UK.

- For psychological disorders, mostly neurotic, an excess in young boys is replaced by an excess in girls by mid-adolescence.

Young people and working adults
- Women have more morbidity from poor mental health, particularly from anxiety and depressive disorders.
- Men have higher rates of schizophrenia and alcohol and drug dependence.
- Women are more likely to consult their GP than men (ratio of 6:4 consultations per year).
- GPs see women more frequently for consultations regarding cancer, obesity, anaemia, migraine, osteoarthritis and back pain.
- GPs see men more frequently for consultations regarding diabetes, heart attacks and angina.
- Women are subjected to a greater number of iatrogenic risks, for example, the oral contraceptive pill and hysterectomies.

Elderly adults
- Osteoporosis is more common in women. The lifetime risk, from the age of 50 years, of fracture of the hip, spine or distal forearm – for which osteoporosis is a major determinant – is 14%, 11% and 13% respectively for women compared to 3%, 2% and 2% for men. The causes of the differences in fracture rates between men and women are not fully understood, but differences in bone density, size and architecture, together with a gender difference in falling, are likely to be major contributors.
- Women have much higher rates of disability than men, especially at older ages. For instance, 80% of men over 85 years were able to go out and walk down the road, compared with just over 50% of women.
- Fourteen per cent of women over the age of 65 years suffer from functional impairments sufficient to require help on a daily basis to remain living in the community, compared to only 7% of men.
- By the age of 85 years and over, these figures have risen to nearly 40% for women and 21% for men.
- Of women over 65 years, 6.4% live in communal homes, compared to 3% of men.

Explaining the inequalities
There are three different explanatory models for understanding the health differences mentioned above:
1. That the differences are due to artefact.
2. That the differences are due to genes or biology.
3. That the differences are due to social causation.

Artefact
Artefact implies that the differences were caused by the method used to collect the data. The suggestion here is that women may self-report more illness because they have a greater awareness of their symptoms and/or less cultural stigma in 'admitting' disease.
   But:
- It has been found by clinical observation that men are more likely to overrate their symptoms (of a cold) in comparison to women – this would lead to an underestimation of differences.

Genetic/biological explanations
Some of the differences have been put down to solely biological factors, for example women may have greater resistance to heart disease because of endogenous female sex hormones. Male babies may be more likely to die than female babies because their lungs tend to be less developed than those of girls of a similar gestation. Furthermore, conditions such as menstruation, pre-menstrual syndrome, morbidity due to pregnancy and childbirth, diseases of the female reproductive organs and the menopause are specific to women. However, while true, this cannot explain the full range of differences in morbidity and mortality between men and women.

Social causation
Social causes highlight the fact that men and women lead very different lives, and social expectations and stereotypes are well established. A few explanations for the observed health differences include:
1. Men lead lives that make them more vulnerable to death from accidents and violence, for example men tend to drive faster.
2. Women may suffer more illness because they undertake more social roles, for example even in couples where both are in full-time employment, women still undertake the majority of domestic work. Women are also more likely to undertake a 'caring' role with regard to their children and spouses.
3. Women are more likely to suffer poverty than men – women tend to be employed in part-time work that pays less, and has fewer benefits, than the kind of employment men typically have.
4. Health-related behaviour also differs between the sexes – until recently, men drank and smoked

more than women. This has resulted in their higher rates of liver cirrhosis and lung cancer. It is expected that the rates of lung cancer will equalize between the sexes now that levels of smoking have.

Ethnic minorities

The Patient's Charter codifies the expectation that those receiving treatment from the NHS can expect their privacy, dignity, religious and cultural beliefs to be respected. The GMC issues guidelines that 'personal beliefs' should not prejudice patient care and that doctors 'must never discriminate unfairly' against patients or colleagues. However, there are noticeable differences in the health status of different ethnic groups. Sociological and epidemiological studies have tried to find out whether these differences arise from biological differences, or whether they are the result of social discrimination.

A brief history of immigration to the UK

The idea of 'race' first appeared in the English language in the early 17th century. However, the idea of race being used as an 'explanation' for differences in observed behaviour only became popular later on. By the mid-19th century the idea that there were 'distinct' races, each with a 'biologically *determined* capacity for cultural development' was etched into the collective consciousness.

Eighteenth-century estimates put the African population in England at 0.2% (mostly slaves), although by the early 19th century this began to decline due to the abolition of slavery. Immigration became an issue later:

- The earliest large-scale migration was probably the post-famine Irish.
- Jewish immigration between the two wars.
- Post Second World War immigration from the Caribbean – in response to labour shortages – many immigrants ended up working for the transport industry or in other low-paid jobs.
- The health service actively recruited from India and Pakistan shortly after its foundation. Thousands of doctors trained overseas immigrated in the 1950s, 60s and 70s. (Of the current 30 000 GPs, about 5000 trained in South Asia, of which 3200 will retire by 2007 leading to an acute GP shortage.)

- In 1962 the Immigration Act placed restrictions on entry into this country.
- East African Asians expelled from Kenya and Uganda in the 70s travelled to the UK – many were professional or business families.
- Modern-day immigration by refugee populations has occurred from Iraq, the Balkans and Afghanistan.
- Ethnic minorities make up approximately 8% of the UK population – the majority of this number are British-born ethnic minorities.
- Ethnic minorities tend to be based in urban environments – often within minority communities. Over half the ethnic population lives in the south-east – forming 20% of Greater London.
- The age and gender distribution of minority ethnic groups is different from the majority population:
  - some minority ethnic groups have more men than women, and all are relatively young
  - Afro-Caribbean and South Asian communities have a higher proportion of households with children than the white population
  - Pakistani and Bangladeshi households are also larger because they are more likely to have three or more adults, whilst Afro-Caribbean households are more likely to be headed by a lone parent.

The health of ethnic minorities

In general, the research carried out in relation to ethnic minorities has focused on immigrants. Part of the reason for this is that death certificates indicate 'place of birth' rather than ethnic group, so the health of those ethnic minorities born in the UK is difficult to study. Key features about the health of immigrant populations include:

1. They tend to show a higher rate of mortality than people born in the UK.
2. They tend to show a lower rate of mortality than those from their home country. (Although the Irish are an exception here.)

The reason for this has been described as the 'healthy migrant' factor – which claims that immigrants tend to be healthier than average for their home population but not as healthy as the population they move into. It has been suggested that the mortality rates are higher than for those born in the UK because they bring with them the risks of

Definitions

Ethnicity – refers to social groups who often share a cultural heritage with a common language, values, religion, customs and attitudes. The members are aware of sharing a common past, possibly a homeland, and experience a sense of difference.

Culture – reflects ethnicity, and refers to habits of thought and beliefs, diet, dress, music, art.

Race – is a construct based on phenotypical biological differences (usually skin colour); social assumptions (often negative) are attributed to biological differences.

Racism – deterministically associates inherent biological characteristics with other negatively evaluated features or actions. Racial discrimination is against the law.

Source: Hillier S 2003

mortality of their earlier life, and then adopt the risks associated with this society.

Mortality

- Ischaemic heart disease accounts for the largest proportion of deaths among men regardless of country of birth.
- Men born in East Africa, the Indian subcontinent and Scotland show higher mortality, and those from the Caribbean lower mortality, compared with the average.
- Cerebrovascular disease was the next major cause of death for men from the Caribbean, West/South Africa and Indian subcontinent.
- Lung cancer was the next main cause of death for Scottish and Irish men, among whom mortality was 46% and 57% higher than the average respectively.
- Irish and Scottish men showed higher mortality from accidents and injuries, and suicides. For both

of these causes, mortality of Scottish and Irish men in class IV/V was more than twice the national rate.

Morbidity

The Health Survey for England – The Health of Minority Ethnic Groups 1999 (Erens 2001) looked in depth at the health of minority ethnic groups – this included minority individuals born both outside and in England. The findings included:

Long-standing and limiting long-standing illness

- Chinese men and women were less likely to report long-standing and limiting long-standing illness than the general population and than all other groups.
- The prevalence of limiting long-standing illness was higher for Pakistani, Bangladeshi and Irish men (35–65% above the general population) and for Afro-Caribbean and South Asian women (20% and 44% above the general population).

Acute sickness

- Chinese men and women were much less likely to report acute sickness than those in the general population and all other minority ethnic groups.

Cardiovascular disease

The survey looked at a range of cardiovascular disease (CVD) conditions – angina, heart attack, stroke, heart murmur, irregular heart rhythm, 'other heart trouble', reported high blood pressure and diabetes:

- For all the above-mentioned conditions with the exception of diabetes, Chinese men and women had lower rates than the general population, and for diabetes the Chinese rates were not significantly higher than those of the general population.
- All South Asian groups showed higher rates than the general population for most conditions, and both Pakistanis and Bangladeshis showed higher rates than Indians.
- Afro-Caribbean men (but not women) had significantly lower prevalence of angina and heart attack than the general population, and both men and women had higher prevalence of diabetes.
- Irish people did not differ substantially from the general population in the prevalence of CVD conditions.
- For some of the main CVD risk factors examined, the differences between people with and without CVD varied within minority ethnic groups and

between these groups and the general population. Risk factors where age-adjusted risk ratios were higher in those with CVD than in those without included raised waist-hip ratio (except Bangladeshi men), overweight/obese (Indian and Bangladeshi women only), and high blood pressure, while risk ratios for cigarette smoking were higher among those without CVD than among those with CVD.

- When all risk factors (such as high blood pressure, cigarette smoking and obesity) were taken into account simultaneously in logistic regression models, the differences in prevalence between each minority ethnic group and the general population were small, and none was significant.

Hypertension

- Compared with men in the general population, mean systolic blood pressures (SBP) were significantly low for Chinese, Pakistani and, in particular, Bangladeshi men.
- Compared with women in the general population, mean SBP were significantly low for Bangladeshi and Chinese women, and high for Pakistani women.
- Pakistani women (risk ratio 1.25) and Afro-Caribbean women (1.21) were significantly more likely to have high blood pressure than women in the general population.
- Within minority ethnic groups, there was no clear and consistent relationship between high blood pressure and either social class or equivalized household income, for either men or women.

Diabetes

- Pakistanis and Bangladeshis of both sexes showed rates over five times higher than the general population and Indians almost three times higher.
- Mortality is three to four times greater in Caribbean-born individuals, three times greater in Asians, and double in African-born individuals.
- Even though Afro-Caribbeans have higher rates of diabetes and hypertension, they have lower cardiovascular disease.

Explanations for variation in cardiovascular disease

1. *Insulin resistance hypothesis*: The association of insulin resistance and heart disease is well recognized. Diabetes and heart disease are both raised above the levels of the general population for Bangladeshi, Pakistani and Indian immigrants. Insulin resistance is associated with patterns of fat deposition – specifically abdominal fat.

However:
- It is not clear that most immigrants from South Asia who have heart disease also have diabetes.
2. *Social stress*: This theory claims that the stress associated with any migration and living with ongoing stressors (such as social deprivation and racism) leads to an increased rate of CVD. It is claimed that the prevalence of CVD across social classes within South Asian immigrants is evidence for this theory.
   However:
- The prevalence of CVD across social classes could be evidence for a biological reason for increased prevalence. Also, if the stress association with migration was responsible, then *all* immigrants would be expected to show raised levels of CVD, but, Caribbean-born men had the lowest rates of CVD – and they are perhaps subject to even more stress (as a population in terms of social deprivation) than South Asian immigrants.

Mental illness

- Highest rates for hospital admissions are from Irish immigrants, followed by Caribbean-born immigrants.
- South Asian immigrants have a lower rate of hospital admission compared to the general population.
- Women are admitted more frequently than men in all immigrant populations except Caribbean populations.
- Admissions due to schizophrenia and paranoia are three times greater for men and twofold greater for women from Caribbean-born populations. This group is also more likely to present to mental-health professionals via the police, or courts, and as a group are *more* likely to be subjected to compulsory detention, compulsory administration of psychotropic drugs and electro-convulsive therapy. This group is *less* likely to be given psychotherapy (or other 'talking' therapies).

Explanations for variations in mental illness

- *Due to 'real' differences* – some people have argued that the stress of migration and the on-going stress of racism leads to increased schizophrenic episodes in Afro-Caribbean populations.
- *Due to misdiagnosis and exaggeration of minor symptoms* – others have claimed that the higher levels of mental illness are due to cultural misunderstanding. Annandale (1998) notes that schizophrenia in Afro-Caribbeans is thought of in

terms of '*threats* to the white community, rather than the *distress* of those who experience mental health problems', and has linked this to a strong 'predisposition on the part of white people in Britain to interpret black people's behaviour as signs of insanity and danger'.

Use of health services
- South Asian and Afro-Caribbean men were more likely than the general population to have consulted their GP in the past two weeks and to have had more than one consultation over this period.
- Among women, contact rates were significantly higher for South Asian and Irish women.
- Relative to the general population, consultation ratios for psychological distress were significantly higher for Irish men (1.5 times) and lower for Chinese men and women (0.59 and 0.41 times) and for Bangladeshi women (0.64 times).
- Relative to the general population, levels of prescribed medicine use by men were low among Chinese men (0.5 times) and high for South Asian men (1.26 to 2.04 times). Indian and Bangladeshi men who had been prescribed medicines were also likely to be taking more drugs per person on medication. Chinese women were low users of medication (0.59), while Bangladeshi (1.37) and Pakistani women (1.42) were relatively high users.
- Afro-Caribbean and South Asian men were two to three times more likely to be on drugs related to the endocrine system. About one-third of drugs dispensed in this group relate to diabetes control.

General explanations for variations in mortality and morbidity
As mentioned before, the inequalities seen in any population, when compared to the general population, can be due to:
1. Artefact.
2. Biological differences.
3. Material differences.
4. Cultural differences.

The inequalities of the ethnic population are probably due to a combination of all of these influences. Artefacts may arise due to the use of census data, which tends to underestimate the size of ethnic populations. Material inequality is common among immigrants; however, with some diseases, such as CVD, where there isn't as steep a gradient across social classes of South Asian immigrants as there is for the ethnic majority population, this may indicate a

biological difference (e.g. increased central obesity and insulin resistance). Finally, cultural differences, such as the 'somatization' of psychological distress in South Asian women, may account for increased GP consultations and reduced diagnosis of mental illness.

Older people

Mortality is related to age. This fact seems self-evident: the older you are, the less life you have to live. However, the relationship between mortality and age is not altogether linear, rather it is a lopsided U-shape – a high rate in the first year (i.e. infant mortality) – a rapid decline and a flat area before rising again in middle age and then a steep rise in older people. Those diseases that are prevalent in the West are predominantly associated with ageing – coronary artery disease and cancer.

However, some sociocultural influences are also thought to affect health:
1. Environmental influences – such as diet, degree of physical activity and smoking, contribute to the diseases of old age.
2. The treatment of older people may lead to their 'disengagement' from social roles – this may be associated with psychological distress such as anxiety and depression, which may, in turn, lead to physical sequelae.

The changing population
During the 20th century, life expectancy rose, and the birth rate fell. These changes have led to an increase in both the absolute number of older people and the proportion of older people within the general population. Older people (i.e. those over 65 years) have been classed as the largest 'dependent' group in society – that is they outnumber children. The word 'dependent' is used because the conventional view is that older people don't work and are, therefore, 'dependent' on the proportion of society that does. This classification is revealing of a generalized view that holds ageing and older people as a 'problem'. This view is being challenged – a Royal Commission on the long-term care of the elderly in 1999 (Sutherland 1999) stated:

> There is now a clear opportunity to see old age for what it is, a stage of life where we have the gift of time to be able to acquire knowledge and experiences for which there may not have been time during working lives. . . . Society should recognise the value inherent in older people, and the value to society in using its ingenuity to

help older people to continue to realise their potential more effectively.

There are good reasons to challenge the idea that old age and older people are problems or threats:

- Many people expect to live 20 or 30 years beyond retirement.
- Only 5% of older people either live in a care home or receive care at home from a local authority.
- While acute health problems (e.g. colds and accidents) do increase with age, they still only affect 20% of males and 25% of females in the very oldest age groups.
- Almost 50% of those over 75 years do not have any illnesses or disabilities that impair their activity level.

However, there are some 'medical' problems of old age. These include:

- Increasing age is associated with a progressive inability to undertake 'activities of daily living'. These include washing oneself, dressing oneself, feeding oneself, climbing stairs and getting to the toilet.
- Multiple pathology – elderly people are more likely to have more than one concurrent medical problem than younger people.
- Polypharmacy – the oldest 16% of the population receives 40% of the drugs. Many elderly patients take more than one type of medication – this can lead to poor compliance (especially if the patient is confused) and a greater number of drug interactions.
- Dementia – only affects 2% of the 65–75 year group, but affects 10–20% of 80+ year olds.
- Use of health services – hospital admissions are greater in older people than in other groups – this is true for most specialties. Older people are also more likely to consult their general practitioner. It has been estimated that the cost of long-term care for older people will rise from £11.1 billion (1995) to £45.3 billion (2051).

Social factors compounding medical problems in older people

Notwithstanding the biological factors that lead to illness in older people, there are social factors as well. These include:

- Poverty:
  - State pensions in the UK are not generous in comparison with the rest of the European Union

  - Older people from social classes IV and V experience more respiratory problems and hypertension compared to older people from social classes I and II
  - Life expectancy at 65 is 2.6 years greater for men from social classes I and II compared to men from social classes IV and V
  - Older people are more likely to be living in poverty compared to the general population. This is especially true of elderly women
  - Poor older people may be less likely to receive some health-care services, or may have poorer health outcomes after receiving these services. For instance, severe visual problems are more likely to remain unrecognized and untreated in older people from low socioeconomic groups.
- Poor housing:
  - Older people tend to live in older housing – this is associated with problems such as increased heating costs and damp. This means that many elderly individuals end up choosing whether to have adequate heating or adequate food. Hypothermia or malnutrition may result.
- Poor mobility:
  - Degenerative disease, such as osteoarthritis, can lead to restriction of access to:
  Goods – an inability to drive may mean that older people are reliant on small local shops. Prices may be higher, and the availability of fresh fruit and vegetables may be reduced.
  Services – such as their GP, may be difficult to attend. Elderly women as a common group require home visits by the GP.
  Social contacts – immobility can hinder the participation of an individual with wider society – this may lead to isolation.
- Fear of crime:
  - This too may restrict the activities of older people – leading to further social isolation.

Ageing and health policy

The ageing population has led to a need for specific health policies on how best to provide for older people. One problem that has beset working out a policy is the question of what demands will be made on the state by the ageing population. Moody (1995) has argued that there are four possible scenarios:

1. *Prolongation of morbidity* – the increase in life years is not accompanied by an increase in quality of life; that is, healthy lifespan is not extended, although absolute lifespan is.

2. *Compression of morbidity* – good health is experienced almost up to the end of peoples' lives, when a 'terminal drop' of health rapidly leads to death.
3. *Lifespan extension* – the healthy lifespan is extended due to advances in medical science and preventative medicine.
4. *Voluntary acceptance of limits* – this scenario aims for the development of a shared 'meaning of old age' which informs views on which health interventions are appropriate (in the sense of being beneficial) and which are futile or merely life-extending.

Sociological views and older people

Higgs (2003) outlines three theories that have been used to account for the position of older people within society:

1. *Disengagement theory*: This American theory claims that old people gradually disengage from a range of social activities and become dependent – unable to fulfil the roles they had previously held. Dependence may be:
   a. financial – receiving a state pension
   b. domestic – needing help to wash, dress, cook or shop
   c. medical – receiving treatment for ill health
   d. social – older parents become less central to the lives of their children as they themselves become parents.

   As people disengage from social roles – especially on retirement – they may experience initial relaxation followed by a period of turmoil, depression and anxiety. This reaction to the loss of status may be similar to the grief of bereavement and has been called *desolation*.

   However, questions have arisen as to whether elderly people choose to disengage or are forced to do so by society.

2. *Structured dependency theory*: This theory stresses the importance of social structures in creating the circumstances elderly people find themselves in:
   a. Financial – the notion of retirement at 65 marks the formal withdrawal from the labour force. In addition, the poverty of older people is a result of poor state pensions.
   b. Labelling and ageism – if older people are seen as 'disengaging' from society and are expected to do so by society, then this becomes a self-fulfilling prophecy. The placement of older people in 'old people's homes' compounds this problem by removing older people from communities – so, in effect, they are 'out of sight and out of mind'.
   c. Cultural emphasis on 'youth' almost by definition excludes older people. The current government has described its approach as 'young, modern Britain', which given the population demographics may be inappropriate.

3. *Third ageism*: This theory is at odds with the previous two, holding that in fact older people are able to enjoy relative good health and affluence. It is pointed out that retirement is forming an increasingly large part of people's lives. There is a blurring between middle age and old age, and older people are increasingly doing those things that were once seen as the younger preoccupations (for example travelling, learning new skills and so on.)

General explanations for health inequalities in older people

Once again it is useful to consider inequalities under the brackets of artefact, biological and social causation. Clearly, biology has a considerable role to play – increasing age is associated with increasing disease. However, this is not the sole cause of health inequalities between young and older people. The elderly are, through a number of mechanisms, deprived of social benefits that help to prevent worsening of health. These include material benefits such as wealth, housing and access to services. In addition to this, there may be cultural issues which lead to older people being less likely to demand health care or support services were they available to them.

- What areas for redress of health inequalities did the Acheson Inquiry highlight?
- What are the aims of the government document *Saving Lives: Our Healthier Nation?*
- What are the categories of the Registrar General's classification of social classes?
- What explanations for health inequalities between social classes did the Black Report consider?
- What explanations for health inequalities between social classes did the Acheson Inquiry consider?
- In what ways could health inequalities between social classes be reduced?
- What is the difference between sex and gender?
- What types of explanation exist for gender inequalities in health?
- What is the difference between race and ethnicity?
- Why do immigrants in general have a higher mortality than people of similar ethnicity who are born in the UK?
- What is the social stress theory?
- What general explanations can be given for variations in mortality and morbidity in ethnic minorities?
- Why do older people have particularly difficult medical problems?

References

Acheson D (Chairman) 1998 An Independent Inquiry into Inequalities in Health Report, London: TSO. Available online at: http://www.archive.official-documents.co.uk/document/doh/ih/ih.htm

Annandale E 1998 The Sociology of Health and Medicine: A Critical Introduction. Cambridge: Polity Press, p. 86

Armstrong D 1989 An Outline of Sociology as Applied to Medicine, 3rd edn. London, Wright, p. 56

Beveridge W 1942 Social Insurance and Allied Services. London: HMSO

Black D, Morris J, Smith C, Townsend P 1980 Inequalities in Health: Report of a Research Working Group. London: Department of Health and Social Security

Department of Health Saving Lives: Our Healthier Nation Cm 4386, 1999 London, HMSO. Available at http://www.archive.official-documents.co.uk/document/cm43/4386/4386-04.htm

Erens B, Primatesta P, Prior G (eds) 2001 The Health Survey for England – The Health of Minority Ethnic Groups 1999. London: The Stationery Office. Available online at: http://www.archive.official-documents.co.uk/document/doh/survey99/hse99.htm

Health Inequalities: Decennial Supplement 1997 London: Office for National Statistics. Available online at: http://www.statistics.gov.uk/StatBase/Product.asp?vlnk=1382&More=Y

Higgs P 2003 Older people, health care and society. In: Scambler G (ed.) Sociology as Applied to Medicine, 5th edn. Edinburgh: Saunders, p. 167

Hillier S 2003 The health and health care of ethnic minority groups. In: Scambler G (ed.) Sociology as Applied to Medicine, 5th edn. Edinburgh: Saunders, p. 146

Marmot M 2003 Understanding social inequalities in health. In: Perspectives in Biology and Medicine 46(3): S9–23

Moody H 1995 Ageing, meaning and the allocation of resources, as reported in Scambler G (ed.) 2003 Sociology as Applied to Medicine, 5th edn. Edinburgh: Saunders, p. 172

Scambler G, Blane D 2003 Inequality and social class. In: Scambler G (ed.) Sociology as Applied to Medicine, 5th edn. Edinburgh: Saunders, pp. 107–23

Sutherland S (Chairman) 1999 With Respect to Old Age: Long Term Care – Rights and Responsibilities. A Report by The Royal Commission on Long Term Care. Available online at: http://www.archive.official-documents.co.uk/document/cm41/4192/4192.htm

Tudor Hart J 1971 The inverse care law. Lancet i; 405–12, as reported by Armstrong D 1989 An Outline of Sociology as Applied to Medicine, 3rd edn. London: Wright, pp. 112–14

Further reading

Scambler G (ed.) 2003 Sociology as Applied to Medicine, 5th edn. Edinburgh: Saunders

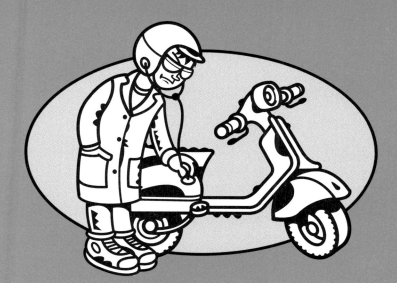

STATISTICS AND EVIDENCE-BASED MEDICINE

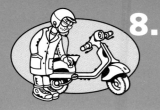

8. Principles of Statistics in Medicine

Introduction

The sheer thought of crunching numbers makes most students go queasy. However, in today's era of medicine, which relies significantly on the correct interpretation of statistics for optimal clinical practice, this chapter seeks to provide a solid base for interpreting data. All that one requires is a basic understanding of algebra, fractions and probability. Most students will have this knowledge as they have studied at least basic mathematics at secondary education level.

Basic concepts

Statistics involves collecting, organizing and interpreting numerical data. It does not simply involve feeding data into a computer in the hope that this will in itself generate a conclusion.

Figure 8.1 outlines some of the terms that are commonly used in any clinical study.

In statistics it is important to understand the term *parameters*. A parameter is a numerical quantity summarizing some aspect of a population of values, e.g. the mean is used to assess the central tendency of

Fig. 8.1 Statistical terms explained.

Statistical terms explained

Statistical term	Meaning
Data	A collection of items of information, e.g. the systolic blood pressure/mmHg of five individuals is 140, 175, 140, 168 and 178 mmHg respectively
Value	The quantity of the variable being assessed, e.g. 175 mmHg is the value of the blood pressure for the second patient
Frequency	The number of times a particular event occurs in a set of data. The frequency with which the value 140 mmHg occurs is 2, since two patients have this value for their systolic blood pressure
Frequency distribution	The resulting output in graphical form showing how the data are distributed
Variable	Any measured characteristic that differs between individuals, e.g. blood pressure. Variables can be qualitative (categorical), e.g. male or female, OR quantitative (numerical): either discrete, in which case the values are whole numbers, as in the case of the number of patients, or continuous, where the data can take any value in the range, e.g. height
Variability	This is a way of summarizing how much individual values in the data vary from each other. It includes terms like variance, standard deviation and range
Population	Do not confuse this with the general meaning of a geographical population. A statistical population is the collection of all possible values of a given variable, e.g. all patient records in a GP practice in London will constitute a population. Often a population will refer to patients both now AND in the future
Sample	A subset of the population on which data are collected. The sample purports to be representative of the underlying population
Random sample	A sample in which each individual/unit has an equal chance of being represented, thus minimizing bias. 'Randomization' usually refers to random allocation in a clinical trial

the data. However, the value of a parameter is rarely known, because we rarely have data available for the whole population. A *statistic* on the other hand is a numerical quantity, e.g. the mean, calculated from a *sample* and used to estimate a parameter.

Averages

Raw data are often unmanageable because of their quantity. Such data can be made more useful by extracting particular information. Hence the use of *measures of central tendency* that assess the location of the middle of the distribution:

The *(arithmetic) mean* is what is generally referred to as the average. It is calculated as follows:

$$\mu \text{ (mean)} = \frac{SX \text{ (sum of all the scores)}}{N \text{ (number of scores)}}$$

For *normal* distributions, the mean is the best measure of central tendency as it is less likely to fluctuate with the sample.

The *median* is the central observation of a set of values, so half the values are above the median and half below it.

The *mode* is the most frequently occurring value in a distribution. It should not be used on its own as it fluctuates with the sample and many distributions have more than one mode (Fig. 8.2).

The *median* is less sensitive to extreme scores than the *mean*. Hence it is a better measure for highly skewed distributions.

Fig. 8.2 Mean, median and mode explained.

The mean, median and mode are identical for symmetric distributions. On the whole, the mean will be higher than the median for *positively skewed* distributions and less than the median for *negatively skewed* distributions.

The measures of spread

The spread of a variable is the *degree* by which the scores on the variable differ from each other (Fig. 8.3). There are several measures of spread: *range, interquartile range, standard deviation, and variance.*

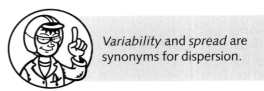

Variability and *spread* are synonyms for dispersion.

Range

This is the simplest measure of spread. It is the difference between the largest and smallest values. It is useful if used as an adjunct to the standard deviation and the interquartile range, but it generally increases with sample size, thereby limiting its usefulness.

Interquartile range

This is calculated as the difference between the 75th percentile (Q3) and the 25th percentile (Q1).

$$IQR = \frac{Q3 - Q1}{2}$$

Its value is not affected greatly by extreme scores, so it is a good measure for skewed data. It is not particularly efficient for normally distributed data.

Mean, median and mode explained

Let us assume that the following is a list of the volume of red blood cells/fl in seven individuals:

86   87   88   89   90   91   92

$$\text{The mean} = \frac{86+87+88+89+90+91+92}{7} = 88.9 \text{ fl}$$

The *median* is 89 fl as it is the central value and there are three values on either side. Had there been eight subjects, e.g.

86   87   88   89   90   90   91   92

the median would have been the mid-point between the two central numbers,

$$\text{so} \quad \frac{89+90}{2} = 89.5 \text{ fl}$$

The *mode* is the most frequently occurring value in the data set (90 fl in this case). When no value in the data set occurs more than once, any and every value is considered a mode.

So to work out the SD, you need to follow these steps:

1. Subtract the mean from each value in turn – this is called the residual.
2. Square each residual.
3. Add all the squared residuals together (this is what the Σ denotes).
4. Divide this figure by n-1 (if you stop here you get the variance – see below).
5. Finally work out the square root of this figure.

Sixty-eight per cent of the data will lie between 1 SD on each side of a normal distribution; 95.4% of the data will lie between 2 SDs and 99.7% between 3 SDs. See Figure 8.4 for a worked example.

Variance (s^2)

Variance is an alternative way of measuring spread. It is equivalent to the standard deviation *squared*, hence it is sometimes abbreviated to s^2. It is used less frequently than the SD as it differs in units from the observations, making comparisons difficult. For example, if the values are originally in ml, the variance will have a value in ml^2.

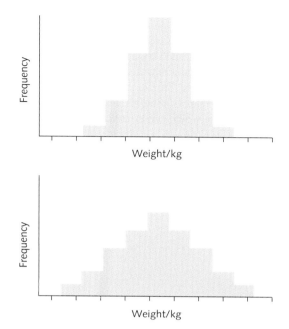

Fig. 8.3 Imagine a situation where two comparable groups of athletes were studied; one was put on a standard diet for several months while the other ate what and when they wanted without control. At the end of the study, their weight distributions could look like this. Both groups have the same mean but differ in spread.

Standard deviation

This is the most commonly used measure of spread. It summarizes an average distance of all the values from the mean of a particular set. The smaller this average distance is, the narrower the spread, and vice versa. It is calculated using the following equation:

$$SD = \sqrt{\frac{\Sigma \left(x_i - \bar{x}\right)^2}{n-1}}$$

Where:
SD is the standard deviation, sometimes represented by the letter 's'
Σ means 'the sum of'
x_i are the observations or values (i indicates all the values of x rather than just one)
$\bar{x}$ is the mean of the values
n is the total number of observations or values.

STANDARD DEVIATION: a worked example Volumes/ml of groups of 10 healthy erythrocytes		
x/ml	$x-\bar{x}$	$(x-\bar{x})^2$
18.4	−0.94	0.884
17.1	−2.24	5.02
18.5	−0.84	0.704
23.2	3.86	14.9
19.6	0.26	0.068
15.4	−3.94	15.5
18.1	−1.24	1.54
20.1	0.76	0.58
23.4	4.06	16.5
19.6	0.26	0.68
Σ = 193.4	Σ = 0.00	Σ = 55.7

$\bar{x}$ = 193.4/10 = 19.34 ml
s^2 = 55.7/9 = 6.18
SD = square root of 6.18 = 2.50 ml
So the correct way of expressing the mean is 19.34 (SD 2.50) ml, which means that about two-thirds (68%) of the groups of 10 cells have volumes between 16.84 and 21.84 ml, which means two thirds of the cells will have volumes between 1.684 and 2.184 assuming the size of erythrocytes follows a normal distribution.

Fig. 8.4 Standard deviation: a worked example.

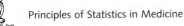
Quantiles

A *quantile* is a way of dividing the total number of observations into equally sized groups where each has the same number of observations. *Percentiles* divide a data set into 100 equally sized groups whereas *quartiles* divide a data set into four equally sized groups. Percentiles are very useful in paediatrics where they help doctors to assess whether the child is growing at the correct rate as indicated by which percentile he/she should be on at that particular age.

The normal distribution

Most *continuous* data can be graphically represented as having a Normal or Gaussian or Bell-shaped distribution. The distribution is fairly symmetrical with scores more concentrated in the middle than around the tails (Fig. 8.5).

Asymmetrical data produce graphical representations which can be said to be *skewed* (Fig. 8.6).

Fig. 8.5 Systolic blood pressure.

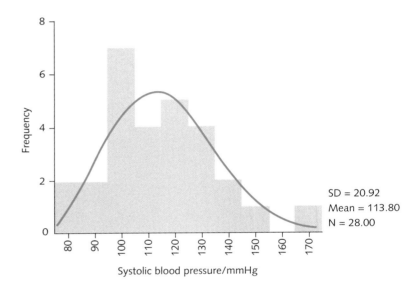

SD = 20.92
Mean = 113.80
N = 28.00

Fig. 8.6 Skewness of data.

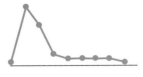

Positive skew – tail stretches to the right

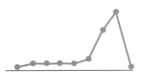

Negative skew – tail stretches to the left

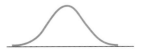

No skew – symmetrical

Precision

In experiments that require us to collect data on a number of subjects, the costs in time and money usually mean that we get only one *sample of the total population* of similar subjects. The standard deviation (SD) of the sub-group gives a statistic that determines the spread of that sub-group. However, often what we would like to know is how variable the means of a number of such samples would be so that we can assess the range over which the mean of the whole population lies without actually taking measurements from the entire population. This is where the *standard error of the mean (SE)* is used.

$$SE = \frac{SD \text{ (standard deviation)}}{\sqrt{N} \text{ (the number of observations)}}$$

The null hypothesis (H$_0$)

This is usually what the investigator seeks to disprove. Say a researcher expects the intake of alcohol to reduce the competence of surgeons; the null hypothesis will be that there is no harmful effect. It allows the researcher to collect the data and to reject the null hypothesis. This is done because it is easier to prove that a hypothesis is false than to prove it is true.

Chance and probability

Chance refers to the likelihood of a particular result happening at random without necessarily describing a general trend. Probability is a measure of the chance of getting some particular outcome. If an outcome is certain, it has a probability of 1. If it is impossible, it has a probability of 0. One of the ways chance is measured in statistics is by using the probability or *P*-value (see section below). *P*-values refer to the probability that an observed statistical difference in any particular sample has occurred by chance.

Sampling distribution

The sampling distribution refers to the distribution of the mean value for a number of samples within a population. It forms a normal distribution with a mean that approximates to the true mean of a population more accurately than any individual sample mean.

The probability value (*P*-value)

One of the most important skills for a clinician is to learn how to analyse the *P*-value. This is the probability of obtaining a statistic which is different from the parameter specified in the null hypothesis. The *P*-value is calculated assuming that the null hypothesis is true (Fig. 8.7). *If the probability value is below the significance level, then the null hypothesis is rejected*.

For example:

H$_0$: There is no difference in the mean peak expiratory flow rate (PEFR) (l/min) of a group of children before and after the administration of a corticosteroid. After calculating the appropriate test statistic using a paired *t*-test, the *P*-value is 0.02. This means that there is a 2% chance that the observed difference in PEFR would have occurred by chance if the null hypothesis was true. Hence, the data provide strong evidence against the null hypothesis and one can conclude that there is a significant improvement in PEFR after taking steroid therapy.

Confidence intervals

To show how much of an effect a treatment actually has, a confidence interval (CI) needs to be calculated. A CI is a range of values that has a specified probability of containing the parameter being measured, e.g. the 95% CI for the mean cardiac output in a group of men can be represented as $4.4 < \mu < 5.2$. This means that the interval between 4.4 and 5.2 has a 0.95 probability of containing the mean, μ, which could be 5 l/min. In practice, calculating CIs is best done with the help of a statistician.

CIs are preferable to *P*-values as they tell one the range of possible effect sizes compatible with the data. They provide different information from that arising from hypothesis tests. Hypothesis testing results in a decision that describes the observed difference of two treatments as either 'statistically significant' or 'statistically non-significant'. The upper and lower bounds of the interval give information on how big or small the true effect might plausibly be. A narrow CI captures only a

---

Steps in hypothesis testing

1. Specify the null hypothesis
2. Select the significance level, usually 5%
3. Calculate the required statistics, e.g. mean
4. Use the appropriate statistical tests
5. Calculate the *P*-value
6. Compare the *P*-value to the significance level
7. Accept/reject the null hypothesis
8. Present your findings in an understandable way!

Fig. 8.7 Steps in hypothesis testing.

small range of effect sizes, and one can be quite confident that any effects far from this range have been ruled out by the study. If the CI is wide, it will capture a diverse range of effect sizes and one can infer that the study size was quite small. Since the study would be 'low-powered', any estimates of the effect size will be imprecise.

However, it is worth remembering that small studies may report non-significance even when there are important real effects. Furthermore, statistical significance does not mean that the effect is real: by chance alone 1 in 20 significant findings will not be genuine.

Type I and II errors

Two kinds of errors can be made when testing significance:

- *Type I* – this occurs when a true null hypothesis gets rejected when in fact it is valid. The probability of its occurrence is called the type I error rate and designated as α. *This is usually set at 0.05 or 0.01*
- *Type II* – this occurs when a false null hypothesis fails to get rejected. The probability of its occurrence is called the type II error rate and designated as *β*

Type I errors are usually more serious than Type II. However, there is a trade-off between the two. The more a researcher protects the experiment against a Type I error, the greater the chance of a Type II error (Fig. 8.8).

Power

The power of a study is the probability of correctly rejecting a false null hypothesis.

If the power of an experiment is low, then the experiment will be inconclusive. There are several methods for estimating power, but these are best

Power = 1 – β (β is the *Type II error* probability)

used by statisticians, hence the need to involve them at an early stage of study design.

Some of the factors that determine the power are the:

- Size of the difference in the outcomes being measured.
- Significance level chosen.
- Variability of data; in particular the size of the standard deviation.
- Distribution of the population – is it normally distributed?

The primary purpose of power analysis is to calculate the sample size. Increasing the sample size increases the power. The more the power, the more accurate the results. However, sometimes it proves too costly and time-consuming to study so many subjects, so a power of about 80% is usually considered satisfactory.

Tests of significance

A probability calculated considering difference in both directions is called a 'two-tailed' probability. However, there are situations where an investigator may only be concerned with difference in one direction. For example, if a new statin is developed, one is only concerned whether it works better than a placebo or not. If its efficacy is not better than that of the placebo, then it will not be used. It does not matter whether or not it is worse than the placebo, so in this case a 'one-tailed' test can be performed. It is easier to reject the null hypothesis with a one-tailed test as long as the effect is in one direction. However, two-tailed tests are more routinely used as they look at both ends of the normal curve and potentially important findings are not missed (Fig. 8.9).

Parametric tests, e.g. *t*-tests, are used to manipulate data based on assumption(s) about the distribution of the data, e.g. normal distribution. Non-parametric tests are also called distribution-free tests and do not rely on the distribution of the data, e.g. the Mann–Whitney *U* test. Sometimes these are less powerful than other tests when the distribution is normal, but might be more powerful when the distribution is greatly skewed.

Remembering Type I and II errors		
Statistical decision	True state of the null hypothesis (H_0)	
	H_0 True	H_0 False
Reject H_0	*Type I error*	Correct
Accept H_0	Correct	*Type II error*

Fig. 8.8 Remembering Type I and II errors.

P-values on either side taken into account

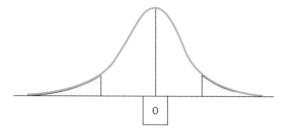

0

Only P-value in the desired direction taken into account

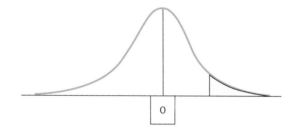

0

Fig. 8.9 One- and two-tailed probabilities.

Correlation

The degree to which two variables are related can be estimated by correlating them. To assess the strength of the linear relationship between the two variables, two methods are used:

1. Pearson Product Moment Correlation or Pearson's correlation – it ranges from +1 to −1. A correlation of +1 means that there is a perfect

positive relationship between the two variables. As the value on the x-axis increases, so does the value on the y-axis. A correlation of −1 implies that there is a perfect negative relationship between the two variables. As the value on the x-axis increases, the value on the y-axis decreases. A correlation of 0 means that the two variables are not related in any linear manner. In practice, the values of the correlation are rarely 0, +1 or −1. Scatter plots are useful in seeing how well the two variables correlate with each other.

2. Spearman Rank Correlation Coefficient or Spearman's *rho* – this differs from (1) above in that mathematical calculations are done only after assigning ranks to the numbers. The smallest value on the x-axis gets a rank of 1 and the ranking increases with the value on the x-axis. The same procedure is followed on the y-axis (Fig. 8.10).

However, it is vital to remember that correlation does not always imply causation. For example, if there was a strong relationship between the number of pubs that have opened in the last ten years and the surgical error rate in trainees, we cannot infer that the pubs are to blame for the surgical errors. Other factors must be taken into account such as lack of practice or the complexity of the procedure.

Prediction and regression

If two variables are closely related, one can predict a person's score on one variable from their score on the second variable with reasonable accuracy. For example, if there is a strong relationship between the forced expiratory volume of air in one second (FEV1) and height, one needs to be able to estimate how much larger the FEV1 measurement will be for a patient SP who is 10 cm taller than

Fig. 8.10 Ranking and calculating variables.

Ranking and calculating variables			
Original x (days)	Ranked x value	Original y (tablets taken)	Ranked y value
7	2	4	1
5	1	7	2
8	3	9	4
9	4	8	3

After ranking the variables, the calculation is the same as for that in the Pearson correlation. In this case, Spearman *rho* = 0.60 and the P-value = 0.40, so within the 95% confidence interval (CI), one can state that any correlation between the number of days and the number of tablets taken is purely coincidental.

patient RT. Assuming that the variables are linearly related, the prediction problem becomes one of finding the straight line that best fits the data. This line is called the regression line and is of the form $y = c + mx$, c = constant/intercept and m= gradient/slope.

Common statistical methods encountered in medicine

All these tests can now comfortably be done on any good statistical package. However, the next few examples are worked out manually so that the reader can understand all the steps involved in generating the statistics (if $P \leq 0.05$, one can reject the null hypothesis, H_0):

1. *t*-tests – should only be used on data that is normally distributed. Furthermore, they are applicable only to *quantitative* measurements that can be summarized by sample means and standard deviations. *t*-tests are a statistical method used on small samples. Because they are small samples they do not have a normal distribution, rather they have the *t*-distribution. The '*t*-value' is a measure of how many SEs the

sample mean lies from the hypothesized, or 'normal,' value. Its interpretation requires the use of a standard *t*-distribution. There are three types:

a. one sample: used to compare a sample mean with a known or hypothesized value where only a single sample of data has been collected

b. independent: used to compare the means of two independent samples as well as measurements of the same variable that have been collected on two different samples of individuals

c. dependent: used to compare the means of two samples of measurements taken on the same subjects or on matched pairs of subjects; repeated measurements of the same variable have been collected on two different occasions on the same individual, or a single set of measurements have been collected on subjects /experimental units that are matched in pairs. This is actually a special case of (a) (Fig. 8.11).

2. Chi-squared tests – used to analyse categorical data (Fig. 8.12).

Fig. 8.11 *t*-tests.

t-tests

One sample *t*-test

In an experiment, the mean PEFR ($\bar{x}$) for 25 asthmatic children was 309.3 l/min and the standard deviation, s = 40.1 l/min. The mean PEFR in the normal population (μ_0) of age-matched children is 328.2 l/min

H_0: The mean PEFR for asthmatic children is equal to 328.2 l/min

$$T = \frac{\bar{x} - \mu_0}{SE} = \frac{309.3 - 328.2}{40.1 / \sqrt{25}} = -2.47$$

Degrees of freedom (d.o.f.) = N − 1 so 25 − 1 = 24

T measures how many standard errors the value of the sample mean lies from the hypothesized value. Looking up this value with 24 d.o.f. on a standard *t*-distribution table indicates that $0.02 < P < 0.05$. Using a statistical package, the exact value of P is 0.021. Hence we can reject H_0.

Independent samples *t*-test

Assume that we divide children into two groups according to how far they live from the main road. Group A ($N_1 = 16$) lives greater than 1 km from the main road and Group B ($N_2 = 15$) lives less than 1 km from the main road. And we want to assess which group has a better PEFR

H_0: There is no difference in mean PEFR between children living near or far from the main road

$$SE\ (\bar{x}_2 - \bar{x}_1) = s_p\ \sqrt{1/N_1 + 1/N_2}$$

$$s_p = \sqrt{\frac{(N_1 - 1)s_1^2 + (N_2 - 1)s_2^2}{N_1 + N_2 - 2}}$$

Fig. 8.11 (*Continued*)

s_1 = SD of sample 1
s_2 = SD of sample 2

$$T = \frac{\bar{x}_2 - \bar{x}_1}{SE\,(\bar{x}_2 - \bar{x}_1)}$$

d.o.f. $N_1 + N_2 - 2$

Assume that for Group A, $\bar{x}_1$ = 319.9 l/min and s_1 = 37.2

And for Group B, $\bar{x}_2$ = 297.9 l/min and s_2 = 41.5

Replacing these values in the above equations gives s_p = 39.3 and T = 1.56 with 29 d.o.f.

Looking up this value on a standard *t*-distribution table, $0.1 < P < 0.5$, so accept H_0

Paired samples *t*-test

Consider 13 children who are invited to the GP clinic to assess whether their PEFR improves after receiving a six-month dose of a new corticosteroid

H_0: The mean change in PEFR after taking the steroid is zero

PEFR (l/min)		
Before treatment	**After treatment**	**Difference**
338	362	24
296	301	5
321	342	21
318	313	−5
279	289	10
249	264	15
332	350	18
277	288	11
246	244	−2
269	280	11
273	314	41
322	330	8
241	228	−13

Mean difference ($\bar{d}$) = 11.08
s (standard deviation of sample) = 13.79
N = 13
T = $\bar{d}$ / SE ($\bar{d}$)
And SE ($\bar{d}$) = s / √N
d.o.f. = N − 1
So substituting all the values gives us T = 2.90 and d.o.f. = 12
Looking up this value on a standard *t*-distribution table, $0.01 < P < 0.02$, so reject H_0

Fig. 8.12 Randomized testing of influenza vaccine.

Randomized testing of influenza vaccine

SR pharmaceuticals has recently launched five vaccines for the immunization against influenza. To test if any are effective, 1350 students from a university agreed to be immunized with the vaccines. The students are randomly divided into five groups of approximately equal size, each group being given a different vaccine. After a few months, student medical records are examined to see who got influenza.

| Type of vaccine | Observed numbers | | | Proportion who got influenza |
| | Number of students | | | |
	Got influenza	Avoided influenza	Total	
I	43	237	280	0.18
II	52	198	250	0.21
III	25	245	270	0.09
IV	48	212	260	0.18
V	57	233	290	0.20
Total	225	1125	1350	0.17

H_0: The proportion of students getting influenza is the same for all types of vaccine. The value of the chi-squared test is calculated as follows:

$$\chi^2 = \frac{\Sigma (O - E)^2}{E}$$

O = Observed number in each 'cell' of the table
E = Expected number in each 'cell' of the table
Σ denotes 'sum over all the cells'

To calculate the *expected number* for each cell, we assume that the null hypothesis is true. We assume that the proportion of all students getting influenza is the same for each vaccine and that this is the same as the overall proportion.

$$\text{Expected number} = \frac{\text{row total} \times \text{column total}}{\text{grand total}}$$

| Type of vaccine | Expected numbers | | | Proportion who got influenza |
| | Number of students | | | |
	Got influenza	Avoided influenza	Total	
I	46.67	233.33	280	0.17
II	41.67	208.33	250	0.17
III	45.00	225.00	270	0.17
IV	43.33	216.67	260	0.17
V	48.33	241.67	290	0.17
Total	225	1125	1350	0.17

We now substitute each observed and expected number into the formula for χ^2:

Fig. 8.12 *(Continued)*

$$\chi^2 = \frac{(43 - 46.7)^2}{46.7} \quad + \quad \frac{(237 - 233.3)^2}{233.3} \quad + \quad \frac{(52 - 41.7)^2}{41.7} \quad + \text{(etc.)}$$

$$= 16.57$$

d.o.f. = (number of columns − 1) × (number of rows − 1)
In this case, d.o.f. = (2 − 1) × (5 − 1) = 4
We then look at a table for percentage points for the *chi-squared* (χ^2) distribution.
$0.001 < P < 0.01$ but using a computer package the exact value of $P = 0.002$
So we reject H_0 and accept that there is a significant difference in the efficacy of the vaccines.

- Discuss the pros and cons of the different measures of central tendency.
- Show how you would assess the variability of a given set of data.
- Explain the roles of confidence intervals in determining the precision of a set of data.
- Discuss the idea of a null hypothesis and the role of *P*-values in its interpretation.
- Outline the importance of power and error calculations before embarking on a study.
- Briefly explain the use of one-tailed and two-tailed levels of significance.
- Describe the concept of 'correlation'.
- Justify the circumstances in which *t*-tests and chi-squared tests would be used in analysing data.
- Compare and contrast the use of odds ratios and relative risks.
- Distinguish between specificity and sensitivity.

Further reading

Davies HTO 2004 What are confidence intervals? Evidence-based medicine. Available online: http://www.evidence-based-medicine.co.uk/ebmfiles/WhatareConfInter.pdf
HyperStat Online Textbook. Available online: http://davidmlane.com/hyperstat

Last MJ 2001 A Dictionary of Epidemiology, 4th edn. New York: Oxford University Press
Swinscow TDV, Campbell MJ 2002 Statistics at Square One, 10th edn. London: BMJ Books

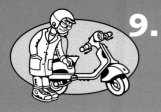

9. Evidence-based Medicine, Research and Clinical Trials

Concepts of evidence-based medicine

Evidence-based medicine is the conscientious, explicit, and judicious use of current best evidence in making decisions about the care of individual patients. It involves much more than just reading research papers. Practising the discipline involves integrating the proficiency and judgement that clinicians acquire over the years with the best available external clinical evidence from systematic research. Excellent doctors will appreciate the value of harmonizing clinical expertise with the best available external evidence. The latter on its own may be inapplicable for an individual patient whilst the former, when used in isolation, results in clinical practice rapidly becoming out of date and decreasing the chance of delivering the best possible patient care.

So why practise evidence-based medicine?

Because it:
- Provides an efficient and systematic way of reviewing vast amounts of medical literature and translating it into good patient care.

- Provides a robust way of managing a disease and enhancing the clinical outcome.
- Serves as a means of modifying current disease-management practices so as to improve the process.
- Can provide a coordinated plan for the management of a disease by the multi-disciplinary team.
- Identifies gaps in the current state of knowledge and highlights areas requiring more investigation.
- Allows one to improve the quality and efficiency of disease-management procedures.

There are some hurdles to practising EBM as well. These include:
- A significant proportion of clinicians lacking formal training in evidence-based medicine and not being able to thoroughly evaluate some research studies.
- Clinicians having the required expertise to analyse the research, but lacking the time to do so.
- Assuming that all that is required to treat a patient is understanding of the anatomical and pathophysiological changes.
- Relying on the fact that it is easier to refer to textbooks, even though they may be out of date.
- Lack of EBM guidelines at the point of practice, e.g. the wards.

Clinical evidence also comes in several levels and its reliability is assessed by the position it occupies in the hierarchy (Fig. 9.1).

Fig. 9.1 Levels of clinical evidence.

Level	Rating	Details
		Levels of clinical evidence
1	* * * * *	Based on randomized-controlled trials (RCTs) or meta-analysis and systematic reviews of such trials. Must be of adequate size to minimize false-positives and false-negatives
2	* * * *	Based on RCTs but of inadequate size. These may show positive results that are not statistically significant or may have a high rate of false-positives and false-negatives
3	* * *	Based on types of study design other than RCTs, e.g. non-randomized controlled or cohort studies, case-controlled studies, case series or cross-sectional surveys
4	* *	Based on the widely accepted and published opinion of respected authorities, expert committees, etc., as presented in consensus conferences or guidelines
5	*	Based on the experience and knowledge of individuals of particular guidelines after peer-discussion

Source: adapted from Journal Club. www.surgical-tutor.org.uk

How to practise evidence-based medicine

This is a systematic and sequential activity as follows:
1. Define an answerable question(s).
2. Locate with maximum efficiency the best evidence, which could include clinical examination, published literature, etc., with which to answer the question.
3. Critically appraise the evidence to assess its validity and usefulness for clinical practice.
4. Implement the results of weighing up the evidence in daily practice.
5. Evaluate the implementation of your findings (this is a form of audit: see Ch. 10).

Study design and interpretation

Epidemiological studies, regardless of type, seek to understand the frequency, pattern and causes of disease in populations. They all permit comparing the experience of disease in terms of time, person or place.

The main types of study-design that one will be confronted with as a clinician are:
- Ecological.
- Cross-sectional.
- Case control.
- Cohort.
- Randomized-controlled trial (RCT).
- Meta-analysis.

Another useful way of classifying the various types of studies is shown in Figure 9.2.

Causal association

Association is the statistical dependence between two variables, i.e. the degree to which the rate of disease in persons with a specific exposure is either higher or lower than the rate of disease without that exposure.

Even the best-designed RCTs have errors, and if errors do not seem to be an obvious explanation for the observed effect, it is still necessary to assess the likelihood that the observed association is a causal one.

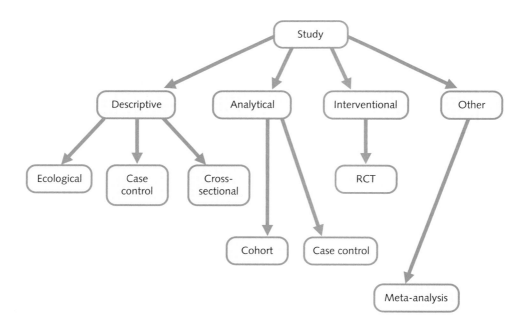

Fig. 9.2 Types of epidemiological studies.

160

Four main areas must be looked at when evaluating a statistical association:

1. Chance – we usually draw inferences about the total population from the sample that we have studied. However, it is unlikely that the estimate from our sample is equal to the estimate in the total population and, in fact, different samples from the same population will yield different estimates due to sampling variation, i.e. just as a result of chance. To assess the effect of chance, we perform appropriate statistical significance tests and calculate confidence intervals.

2. Bias – leads to an incorrect estimate of the effect of an exposure on the development of a disease or outcome of interest. There are different types of bias:

   a. selection bias – occurs when there is a systematic difference between the characteristics of the people selected for a study and the characteristics of those who were not, e.g. all patients who enrol for an exercise ECG experiment will probably be health conscious

   b. measurement or information bias – occurs when measurements or classifications of disease or exposure are inaccurate and do not measure correctly what they are supposed to measure. Errors in measurement may be introduced by the *observer* (observer bias), by the *study individual* (responder bias), or by the *instruments* (e.g. questionnaire or sphygmomanometer) used to make the measurements. Observer bias can also occur if a doctor tends to favour a particular treatment. For example, a doctor may judge the outcome for the patients undergoing a new treatment in a more favourable way than for those in a placebo group. *Recall bias* occurs when patients' recall of their past exposure to risk factors differs from the recall of the controls. If patients with breast cancer are more likely to remember having ever used oral contraceptives than healthy controls, a spurious association between oral contraceptives and breast cancer will result.

3. Confounding – occurs when an estimate of the association between an exposure and the disease is mixed up with the real effect of another exposure on the same disease – the two exposures being correlated. For example, a report was published that made the claim that coffee consumption is associated with the risk of cancer of the pancreas. The importance of this association was disputed because it was pointed out that coffee consumption was correlated with cigarette smoking, and cigarette smoking was known to be a risk factor for pancreatic cancer. Therefore, smoking confounded the association between coffee and cancer of the pancreas. For a variable to be a confounder, it must be associated with the exposure under study and it must also be independently associated with disease risk in its own right (Fig. 9.3).

4. Cause – *The Bradford Hill Criteria, 1965* are pivotal in identifying a causal relationship between two variables (Fig. 9.4).

In epidemiology, it is rare that one study alone will provide sufficient proof that a certain exposure affects the risk of a particular disease. However, the degree of one's belief in the association will depend on the type of study design.

3Cs and a B to establish the association between two variables are **C**hance, **C**onfounding, **C**ause and **B**ias.

Choosing the study design

Spending adequate time on designing a study will save the investigator having to deal with problems during the running of the study. So the study must:

- Directly answer your research question.
- Have adequate power.
- Have ethical approval.
- Be well-budgeted as patient recruitment and assessment can be expensive.
- Allow for good randomization and blinding, if applicable.
- Be valid; this can be achieved by minimizing bias and confounding.

Types of study
Ecological study
Ecological studies use groups or populations rather than individuals as units of observation. They include studies of geographical differences and time trends in disease incidence and prevalence. While ecological studies provide useful information on exposure,

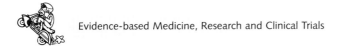

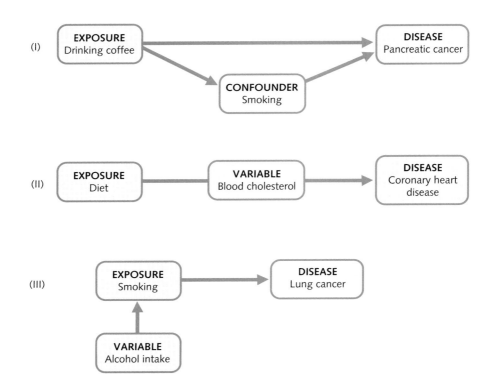

Fig. 9.3 Associations
In these examples, only (I) is a confounding variable. In (II), the variable is intermediate in the causal path between the exposure and the disease. In (III), the variable is associated with the exposure under study but is not independently associated with the disease.

Fig. 9.4 Bradford Hill Criteria (1965).

Bradford Hill Criteria (1965)	
Criteria	Details
Temporal relationship	Exposure must precede the disease
Plausibility	Results must be consistent with other knowledge, e.g. animal experiments, biological mechanisms, etc.
Consistency	There should be other studies that replicate the results of the study in question
Strength	Measured by the magnitude of the relative risk. Stronger associations are more likely to be causal
Dose–response relationship	If increasing levels of exposure lead to increasing risks of disease, the higher the chance of causality
Specificity	If a particular exposure increases the risk of a certain disease but not the risk of other diseases, then this is strong evidence in favour of a cause–effect relationship
Reversibility	When the removal of a possible cause results in a reduced disease risk, the likelihood of the association being causal is strengthened

162

disease and modifying factors, they are in most cases inadequate to establish causal relationships. An example of such a study would be one that compares the incidence of skin cancer for people living at different latitudes.

Cross-sectional studies
Describes the distribution of a disease in relation to:
- Person (age, sex, race, marital status, occupation, lifestyle).
- Place (variation between and within countries).
- Time (variation over time and season).

Advantages include:
- Quick and easy.
- Relatively cheap and easy to carry out.
- Useful for health-care providers to allocate resources efficiently and plan effective prevention.
- Providing clues leading to hypotheses that can be tested in analytical studies.
- Status of individuals with respect to absence or presence of both exposure and disease assessed at *the same point in time*.

Disadvantages include:
- Hypothesis is generally poorly defined.
- Confounding is high and hence it is difficult to prove causality.
- Cannot distinguish whether exposure preceded disease.
- Selection and recall bias.

An example of a cross-sectional study would be studying the different reasons for people consulting their GPs in three different cities by using a cross-section of the individual populations in the three cities.

Case-control study
A case group with disease is compared with a control group without disease and the proportion of exposure in each group is compared.

Advantages include:
- Quick and inexpensive.
- Well-suited for evaluation of diseases with long latent periods.
- Optimal for evaluation of rare *diseases*.
- Can examine multiple aetiological factors for a single disease.
- Can use expensive tests.
- Measurement consistency as exposure and disease collected at the same time.

Disadvantages include:
- Inefficient for evaluation of rare *exposures*.

- Cannot compute incidence rates in exposed and unexposed individuals.
- The temporal relationship between exposure and disease may be difficult to establish.
- Problems with recall and selection bias.
- Cannot estimate the incidence of disease.

An example of a case-control study would be the occurrence of eosinophilia-myalgia syndrome (EMS), and the previous use of a specific brand of L-tryptophan.

Cohort studies
Subjects are classified according to presence or absence of exposure to one or more factors and followed for a specific time period to determine the development of disease. There is a follow-up period of several years to allow an adequate number to develop the outcome.

Advantages include:
- Valuable for rare exposures.
- Can examine multiple effects of a single exposure.
- Can elucidate temporal relationship between exposure and disease.
- Minimize bias in exposure ascertainment.
- Allow direct incidence calculation.

Disadvantages include:
- Inefficient for evaluation of rare diseases.
- Prospective: expensive and time-consuming.
- Retrospective: availability of adequate records.
- Losses of follow-up can affect results.

Prospective and retrospective cohort studies
- The choice of study type (prospective or retrospective) depends upon whether the outcome of interest has occurred at the time the investigator initiates the study.
- Prospective cohort study: exposure may or may not have occurred but disease has not occurred yet.
- Retrospective cohort study: investigation initiated after both exposure and disease have occurred.
- Cohort study can start retrospectively by defining cohort and exposures and then follow-up cohort (for example, congenital malformations and later cancer).
- Retrospective cohort studies are cheaper and thus better for diseases with a long latency.
- Retrospective studies require information from pre-existing records (confounder information may be missing).

An example of a cohort study would be dividing 100 000 doctors into four cohorts: non-smoker, light, moderate and heavy smoker, and following them for ten years to assess their causes of death. The idea is to show that the more you smoke, the greater your chances of acquiring lung cancer.

Randomized-controlled trial

Randomized-controlled trials (RCTs) are clinical studies in which two or more forms of care are compared and the participants are allocated to one of the forms of care in the study in an unbiased way. It is the gold-standard for evaluating the evidence from clinical research. Additional features include single or double-blindedness and/or placebo-controlled.

Advantages include:
- Equal distribution of influential variables.
- Blinding more likely – either double-blind or single-blind.
- Randomization facilitates statistical analysis.
- Placebo-controlled preferable, but not always possible.

Disadvantages include:
- Expensive: time and money.
- Volunteer bias (Fig. 9.5).
- Ethically problematic at times.

An example would be a double-blind RCT evaluating the efficacy of cetirizine versus placebo in reducing the symptoms of seasonal allergic rhinitis.

Systematic review

This involves the whole process of finding, appraising and synthesizing the relevant evidence. A meta-analysis is just the number-crunching aspect of a systematic review.

Advantages include:
- Gives a clearer picture by combining the current pool of evidence.

- Precise.
- Overcomes bias.
- Transparent as good systematic reviews will tell you what assumptions were made.

Disadvantages include:
- Location and selection of studies to be included may be poor.
- The different studies are heterogeneous and some good ones can be combined more easily with each other than with poor ones.
- The patient groups studied, the outcomes measured and the interventions used may differ in the individual studies so how does one combine two different outcomes?
- Some important data will have to be discarded from individual studies as it will not be found in other studies.
- Conflicts with novel experimental data, which should be included in the meta-analysis with caution.
- Publication bias.

An example would be a meta-analysis of RCTs assessing whether laparoscopic or open groin hernia repair is better.

Measures of association between exposure and disease

The basic aim of epidemiological research is to investigate the association between exposure to a risk factor (e.g. smoking) and the occurrence of disease. This requires that the incidence in a group of persons exposed to the risk factor be compared with a group not exposed. There are two ways of doing this, *relative risk* and *attributable risk*.

Effect of bias and confounding on different types of studies					
Probability of:	Ecological	Cross-sectional	Case-control	Cohort	Randomized trial
Selection bias	N/A	medium	high	low	low
Recall bias	N/A	high	high	low	low
Loss to follow-up	N/A	N/A	N/A	high	medium
Confounding	high	medium	medium	low	very low

Fig. 9.5 Effect of bias and confounding on different types of studies.

Relative risk

$$\text{Relative risk} = \frac{\text{Incidence in the exposed group}}{\text{Incidence in the unexposed group}}$$

The *relative risk* can either be calculated using the *cumulative incidence*, in which case it is sometimes referred to as the *risk ratio*, or calculated using the *incidence rate*, when it may be referred to as the *rate ratio*.

The relative risk is used as a measure of aetiological strength. A value of 1.0 indicates that the incidence of disease in the exposed and the unexposed is identical and thus the data show no association between the exposure and the disease. A value greater than 1.0 indicates a positive association or an increased risk among those exposed to a factor. Similarly, a relative risk less than 1.0 means there is an inverse association or a decreased risk among those exposed, i.e. the exposure is protective.

Attributable risk

Information on the relative risk alone does not provide the full picture of the association between exposure and disease.

The *attributable risk* is a measure of exposure effect that indicates on an absolute scale how much greater the frequency of disease in the exposed group is compared to the frequency in the unexposed group, assuming that the relationship between exposure and disease is causal. It is the *difference* between incidence in the two groups.

It can either be calculated using the *cumulative incidence*, in which case it is sometimes referred to as the *risk difference*, or calculated using the *incidence rate*, when it may be referred to as the *rate, difference*.

The *attributable risk* is especially useful in evaluating the impact of introduction or removal of risk factors. Its value indicates the number of cases of the disease among the exposed group that could be prevented if the exposure were completely eliminated. In RCTs, attributable risk is referred to as 'absolute risk reduction'.

$$\text{Attributable risk} = \text{Incidence in the exposed} - \text{Incidence in the unexposed}$$

Odds ratio

Relative risk can be calculated from cohort studies, since the incidence of disease in the exposed and non-exposed is known. In *case-control studies*, however, the subjects are selected on the basis of their disease status (sample of subjects with a particular disease [cases] and sample of subjects without that disease [controls]), not on the basis of exposure. Therefore, it is not possible to calculate the incidence in the exposed and non-exposed individuals. It is, however, possible to calculate the *odds of exposure*. This is the number of people who have been exposed divided by the number of people who have not been exposed. The *odds ratio of exposure* is the *odds of exposure* in the cases divided by the *odds of exposure* in the controls (Fig. 9.6).

$$\text{Odds ratio} = \frac{\text{Odds of exposure in the diseased group (cases)}}{\text{Odds of exposure in the disease-free group (controls)}}$$

It can be shown that this *odds ratio* of exposure is generally a good estimate of the relative risk if the disease is rare.

Pharmacological research

The aim of pharmaceutical research and development is to create new medicines to meet medical needs and:

- Establish their safety and efficacy.
- Develop reliable ways of manufacturing products with consistent high quality.
- Generate knowledge of how to use the new product to the best effect (Figs 9.7, 9.8).

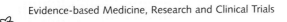

Fig. 9.6 Summarizing the relationship between binary variables.

Summarizing the relationship between binary variables

We conduct a study on pravastatin alone versus pravastatin and dieting for the reduction of cholesterol and measure the mortality of patients after five years. The results are as follows:

	Death	No death	Total
Pravastatin (control group)	49	26	75
Pravastatin and dieting (experimental group)	35	41	76

- In the pravastatin group, risk = 49/75 = 65% = 0.65 = P1
  In the pravastatin and dieting group, risk = 35/76 = 46% = 0.46 = P2

- Absolute risk reduction (ARR) = control risk − experimental risk
  Used to contrast between different therapies
  ARR = 0.65 − 0.46 = + 0.19 (a positive sign shows that the experimental group shows some benefit whilst a negative sign shows that the experimental treatment appears to be doing harm)

- Relative risk (RR) = P1/P2 = 0.65/0.46 = 1.41 and since this is greater than 1, it means that the risk of dying in the control group is higher whereas if the figure were less than 1, it would mean that the risk of death in the control group would be lower

- Relative risk reduction (RRR) = (P1 − P2)/P2 = (0.65 − 0.46)/0.65 = 0.37
  This means that the patient who is on the dieting and drug regime is at an approximately 37% lower risk of experiencing an adverse event relative to the risk of a patient in the drug-only group

- Odds ratio (OR) $= \dfrac{P1/(1 - P1)}{P2 / (1 - P2)} = (0.65/0.35) / (0.46/0.54) = 2.18$

  So a patient on the experimental treatment is half as likely to die as a patient on pravastatin alone

- From the ARR, we can say that 19 adverse events were prevented in every 100 patients (0.19 = 19%) who were on the dieting and drug regime
  So the number needed to treat (NNT) = 100/19 = 5.26 patients, which means that six patients would be treated for every adverse event
  When the new therapy is harmful, we would calculate the number needed to harm (NNH) in the same manner for the NNT, the only difference being that our ARR value would be negative

Fig. 9.7 Phases of clinical development.

	Phases of clinical development	
Phase	Actions	Approximate number of patients
Pre	Compound acquisition and animal testing	N/A
I	Pharmacology and toxicology on human volunteers: • first administration to man • tolerability • pharmacological and pharmacokinetic effects	20–80
II	Uncontrolled treatment-effect studies on patients: • efficacy • dose-ranging • relative safety	100–200
III	Randomized-controlled trials: • confirmation of dose • efficacy in specific indications • use in specific populations • adverse events/safety data	1000–3000
IV	Post-market surveillance: • supplement of phase III • new indications/populations • new presentations • adverse events • long-term benefits	N/A

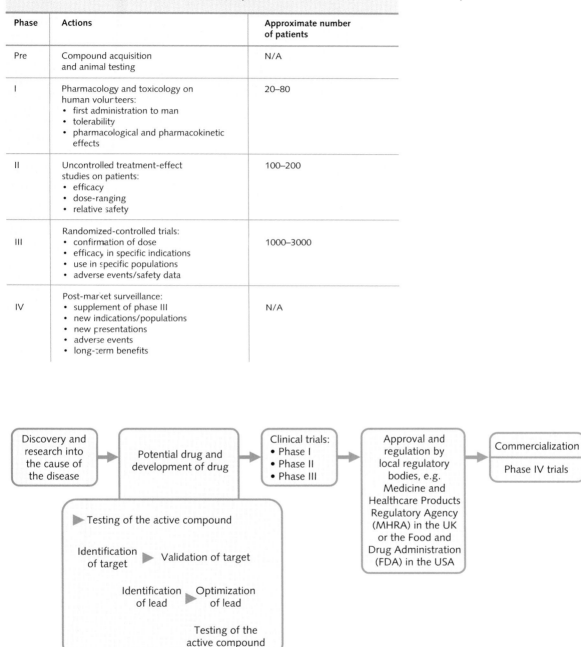

Fig. 9.8 From molecule to marketplace.

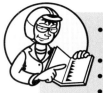

- Discuss the importance of evidence-based medicine (EBM) in the daily practice of the modern clinician.
- Describe the different stages in effectively practising EBM.
- Contrast the various types of epidemiological studies.
- Outline the criteria for establishing a causal relationship between two variables.
- Discuss the steps involved in designing a potential drug.

Further reading

Bhopal RS 2003 Study design. In: Bhopal RS (ed.) Concepts of Epidemiology. New York: Oxford University Press, pp. 231–65

Centre for Evidence-Based Medicine, University Department of Psychiatry, Warneford Hospital, Headington, Oxford OX3 7JX 2004 Study design. Oxford Centre for Evidence-Based Medicine. Available online at http://www.cebm.net/study_designs.asp#random

Davies HTO, Cromie IK 2004 Evidence-based medicine. Hayward Medical Communications, a division of Hayward Group plc. Available online at http://www.evidence-based-medicine.co.uk

Greenberg RS et al. 2001 Medical Epidemiology. Lange Medical Series, 3rd edn. New York: McGraw-Hill, pp. 91–139

Greenhalgh T 2003 Why read papers at all? In: Greenhalgh T (ed.) How to Read a Paper – The Basics of Evidence-based Medicine, 2nd edn London: BMJ Books, pp. 1–14

Sackett DL, Rosenberg WMC, Gray JAM, Haynes RB, Richardson WS 1996 Evidence-based medicine: what it is and what it isn't. British Medical Journal 312: 71–2

Swinscow TDV, Campbell MJ 2002 Statistics at Square One, 10th edn. London: BMJ Books

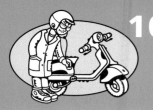
What is audit?

The nightmare happens at interview '. . . can you tell us what you understand by the term audit?' Before you have palpitations, let us look at the political jargon.

Start by thinking of the overriding theme:

> Audit is the process of reviewing the delivery of health care to identify deficiencies, so that they may be remedied
>
> (Crombie and Davies 1993)

- The principal aim of audit is to improve the quality of medical care.
- Audit looks at how a service ought to be delivered.
- It then compares that to the way it is currently being delivered.

The concept was introduced in the government's White Paper for the NHS *Working for Patients* (1989), and since the early 1990s it became a contractual requirement for doctors in the hospital setting.

Audit is a hot topic at interview. Have a two-sentence definition that you could expand on if they push you, for example:
  Audit is central to clinical governance and is a mechanism for improving patient care. It is a cycle of comparing actual practice with pre-agreed standards or guidelines.

A health-care professional's aim is to do the best for an individual patient, within the available resources, by addressing the particular needs of that patient.

In the past there were no agreed standards as to what care the patient with a given illness or condition might expect from the NHS. As a consequence there were no reference points against which one could assess and evaluate the quality of clinical care given.

Audit incorporates a structure in which standards are set and then practical solutions are found to bring that service up to a particular standard.

A 'standard' in a clinical audit describes 'what should be done' in a particular clinical situation. It must be up to date and be based upon sound research evidence. It is a statement that explicitly lays out (in precise, definite and measurable terms) the quality of care expected.

Another way of looking at audit is:
  A cycle of setting standards, monitoring performance, and implementing change to bring performance up to standard (Healy 1998).

In essence audit is a review process that *monitors clinical quality* (in a similar way that industries use quality control checks) to ensure that all the energies going into ' intervention X' are as effective as possible, and are not departing from agreed standards of care.

So audit is central to all our professional lives – it is a powerful tool that helps us to practise medicine to the *best standard*. It is also meant to be a non-threatening exercise for all those involved in it.

However, in order for an audit to be successful, health-care professionals must be receptive to the possibility that their and the team's clinical practice (and thus the quality of their treatment and care) may in fact be improved.

Although patient care is the focus of audit activities, it is also an essential mechanism (as part of clinical governance) for the medical profession and

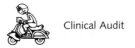
government to move from a 'culture of blame and scapegoating' to achieving an atmosphere where *quality of care* is the focus, i.e. learning from our mistakes – what works well, what does not and making necessary improvements (Fig. 10.1).

What areas can an audit focus on within the NHS?
- Regional variations in the delivery of health care ('postcode lottery').
- The use of limited resources (cost-effectiveness).
- Deficiencies in care delivered (improving outcomes).
- Technological advances (how technology is being used).
- Medical education (the process is an educational tool – review and reflection).
- It *can* act as a political tool (e.g. to argue for more resources).

Audit can look at many levels of services, for example:
- Individual treatments or investigations in a specific hospital.
- Departmental performance.
- Regional or trust performance compared with national levels.

Society is continuously watching the practice of health-care professionals. This is shown by the rise in demands of pressure groups, press coverage and litigation. Audit helps us to improve our practice of medicine and maintain the respect and appreciation of our patients.

Why should I learn about it?

Clinical audit is a topic that comes up regularly at interview – even if you haven't completed any audits, you are expected to have a working understanding of them.

It is increasingly becoming desirable to have an audit under your belt for obtaining junior-grade posts (e.g. SHO training programmes) and often a pre-requisite for middle-grade (specialist registrar) posts. So not only is it good for the patient, but it is also good for your career!

All specialties hold audit meetings (which include mortality and morbidity meetings) and both as a student and as a junior doctor it is advisable to understand the basic processes.

Audit is one of the cornerstones to clinical governance. Both have become hot political topics, and are at the centre of the current NHS reforms: 'The NHS Plan'. It is also strongly promoted by the National Institute of Clinical Excellence (NICE). Therefore, it is key public policy and greatly relevant to the future of the NHS and your working environment.

Audit vs. research

Confusion often arises between research and audit. Audit is a separate concept from research. Both

Fig. 10.1 Key features of an audit.

Key features of an audit

- The aim of audit is to improve quality of care
- Audit involves setting 'standards' and measuring against them
- It examines clinical issues (diagnosis, treatment and patient care)
- Audit involves changing our everyday practice to remedy any deficiencies
- This improves patient outcomes
- The process should be led by clinicians (not academics or management)
- It is a team effort with multi-disciplinary involvement

involve measuring patient outcomes and, although for different purposes, they both have important roles in clinical governance.

Figure 10.2 highlights the differences between audit and research. In summary:

- We use research to seek out new information which provides the foundation for agreeing what we should be doing, i.e. it gives us the evidence we need upon which to base our standards.

- Audit examines current practice to see if we are maintaining the standards we have set for ourselves.

The audit cycle

Audit is a process with discrete stages (Fig. 10.3); however, it is also a continuous exercise, as shown in Figure 10.4.

The differences between research and audit

Research	Audit
Sets standards	Maintains standards
Seeks new knowledge	Tests conformity with tested knowledge
Defines what best practice is	Asks if best practice is being implemented
What is good care?	Is good care being practised?
Aims to increase knowledge	Aims to improve outcomes

Fig. 10.2 The differences between research and audit.

The essential stages of a clinical audit

- Setting a 'standard of care' (i.e. evidence base)

- Assessment by audit (measuring what is currently done)

- Comparing current practice with the 'standard of care'

- Implement change (alter any deficient practices)

- Audit to make sure things have actually improved ('closing the loop')

Fig. 10.3 The essential stages of a clinical audit.

Fig. 10.4 Medical audit cycle. Modified from Fowkes FGR. Medical Audit Cyde. *Med Educ* 1982; 16: 228–38.

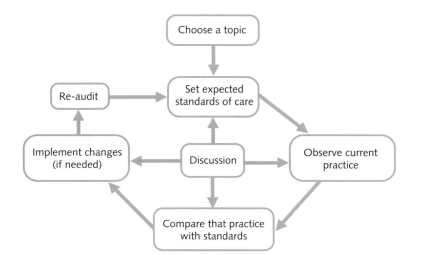

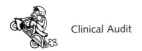

Choosing a topic

All aspects of medical care are suited to audit and there are an abundance of topics from all specialties. When considering a topic, you may be responding to an identified problem or to new evidence.

The elements to take on board are:

- Is the area of interest of high cost, volume, or risk to staff or users?
- Do you have the time and resources to complete the audit cycle?
- Is the project supported by those who have the authority and commitment to put changes into practice?
- Will looking at this area help to improve the quality of patient care?

Ultimately, the only reason for doing audit is to effect change. Without change, it will just become another report or inquiry which gathers dust on the shelves.

> The problem audited should be capable of change and if successful the change should be worthwhile
> (Crombie and Davies 1993)

Setting standards

As discussed before, a standard describes 'what should be done' in a particular clinical situation. Standards are the hallmark of audit and the basis of measurement against which we judge a service. However, identifying a standard is arguably the most difficult part of the audit.

The standard should correspond to the specific aims and objectives of your audit; it may come from:

- National standards – such as set by NICE, a Royal College or a professional body.
- Regional standards – e.g. agreed levels of care set across an NHS trust.
- Locally adapted standards – a national standard tailored to your department.
- There may be no standard – in which case you must set one.

To set your own standards requires considerable effort, but can be ultimately more rewarding. It will be specific to your environment and adaptable to local circumstances. In order to set a new standard, there must be a negotiation both within the audit group and with service deliverers. This will mean that it will be more acceptable to everyone and there will be a sense of ownership.

Firstly, where to look for evidence:

- A literature search (to see what evidence there is).
- Comparison with other centres (i.e. is there a geographical variation in outcomes between you and another centre).
- Clinical experience (if there is no evidence in that area – an estimation of what level of care should be achieved).
- A consensus to be reached, between all the teams and individuals concerned within that area of patient care.

Secondly, phrasing a standard. Crombie and Davies (1993) define a standard as having three parts:

1. The setting of 'criteria'
   a. This sets the point at which good care ends and inadequate care begins.
   b. It is a clinically relevant variable, which is easily defined and measured

e.g. a random glucose of <10 mmol/l for a Type 1 diabetic patient.

2. Outlining a 'target'
   a. The proportion of patients who should meet this criterion.
   b. A target is essential as some patients will not comply, treatment will fail, etc.
   c. It must be a compromise between clinical importance, attainability (i.e. must be realistic) and acceptability (to all the team).
   d. Set too high, the target becomes impossible and you have **created** a health-care problem. Set too low, and we are not striving for the best medicine, but convenient medicine.

e.g. 85% of Type I diabetics should have a glucose of <10 mmol/l. In our example, the random glucose is relevant because it indicates good diabetic control; it is evidence-based because there is published evidence to suggest that it will decrease the risk of diabetic complications (e.g. nephropathy); it ought to be achievable for the majority of diabetic patients and it

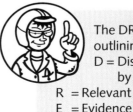

The DREAM acronym for outlining a target:
D = Distinct, i.e. not covered by other items
R = Relevant
E = Evidence based
A = Achievable
M = Measurable.

is clearly measurable. It is distinct as long as you are not concurrently measuring glycosylated haemoglobin.

3. Defining 'allowable exceptions'
   a. Situations in which the criteria do not apply to certain patients
   e.g. If the patient has a concurrent illness at the time of measurement. So in this example our standard of care is that: 'An acceptable random blood glucose measurement is less than 10 mmol/l in a Type I diabetic patient. We aim that 85% of the population will attain this, UNLESS they have a concurrent illness at the time of measurement.'

Irrespective of who set the standard – NICE or John Smith of Any Town Hospital Trust – a standard must convey to everyone (clinicians, auditors and patients) precisely what is expected from the service and what it is being measured against. The standards used should be included in any audit report as they are what we have measured the service against.

Assessment in audit

By this, we mean the observation of current practice, and the collection of data. There are different ways of carrying out an audit cycle, and these can vary in complexity from looking at one subset of patients to multi-centre analysis of all patients seen.

Data collection is of course an essential part of the cycle, as without data we cannot hope to know what to change or how.

It must be broken down into manageable steps:
- Decide where your data are coming from:
  – Is it prospective (collecting new data) or retrospective (getting information from routine sources)?

– What will be the sources of the data?
– Who will collect the data?

There are two ways to collect data, and the method will depend on which source of information you use (Fig. 10.5):

1. Retrospective audit uses information which is routinely kept by your organization (e.g. waiting times, blood results, patient outcomes). The information should be readily available, accurate and complete (e.g. patients' medical notes, biochemistry results).

2. Prospective audit allows you to set up a reporting system where no such data collection exists (e.g. what time the patient ate or why their discharge was delayed).

- Select an audit sample:
  – The important question is: what sample will be sufficient for senior colleagues to agree that they will introduce changes if the audit indicates the need for this?
  – Think about age, aspect of service and time period
  – Ensure the sample is free from selection bias.
- Create a pro forma (data collection form):
  – The data collected must evaluate every aspect laid out in the standard
  – The questions asked are crucial to successful audit
  – Make sure your data collection sheet is asking the right questions, in a relevant way
  – Remember to keep all data confidential (preferably anonymous), though identifiable to the auditors
  – Use as few words as possible

Fig. 10.5 Audit time spans.

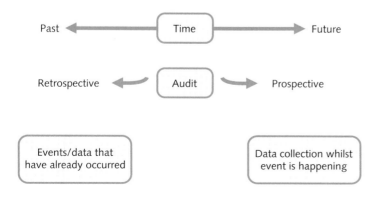

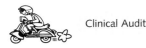

- Free text is difficult to analyse and should be avoided.
- Trial a pilot audit on a small sample of patients:
  - Sounds boring but can save a lot of heartache
  - Undertake a mini-audit on a very limited number of patients (e.g. five) to check that: the questions are not ambiguous, the information is answering your questions and that the data are not too difficult to obtain from the record.
- Carry out the audit – you are ready to begin.

Comparing current practice with the standard (data analysis)

At the end of the assessment section of the audit, there will be three sets of data:
1. Those that conformed to the standard.
2. Those that didn't conform BUT that fitted the exceptions.
3. Those that didn't conform to the standard OR meet the exceptions.

Each should be reported, and you must calculate whether you have met your target or not, for each standard criterion.

At this stage it is important to have a consensus meeting where you formally present your data to senior colleagues and all the interested members of the health-care team and patient consumer groups.

Implementing change

This is the final step in the loop, and provides the reason for the whole exercise. By identifying the areas that are not living up to the prescribed level of care, we can start to think of ways to ameliorate the problem.

The aim of audit is to improve the delivery of health care, so there is no point in simply describing a health-care problem.

Unfortunately, it is usually far easier to identify a deficiency than to solve it overnight. Whilst some problems (such as lack of staff or insufficient training on technique X) may be relatively straightforward to correct, there are many subtle barriers and underlying causes that make effecting change difficult. For example, it may involve more work for the provider of that service with no extra resources or it may be very different from conventional practice and, therefore, seem challenging.

This is a crucial phase, as it offers the possibility for practical solutions to be forged. Therefore, it should be a decision, guideline or change in which all

staff involved are consulted for an opinion. Changes must be implemented with care and incrementally so as not to disrupt the status quo unnecessarily. It should also be explained to staff not directly involved in making the decision why it has been made and stressed that it is hoped that it will lead to improved patient care.

Closing the loop: re-audit

It is too easy to assume that we have effected great change by our efforts. Since audit is intended to improve patient care, we must re-audit (close the loop) in order to assure ourselves that the solution we have implemented has had an impact upon the original problem.

Within management circles and NHS publications, one phrase crops up repeatedly:

The basic principle of audit is that it should be 'complete, accurate, transparent and honest'

This should be reproduced in any exam question on audit as there is likely to be a mark for saying it!

Other characteristics of audit

Confidentiality

A central part of audit is confidentiality – not only due to those whose care has been reviewed (GMC guidance, The Data Protection Act 1998, The Human Rights Act 1998) – but also due to the medical staff who managed them. Audit will only blossom where individuals are confident that the findings (which may include individual failings) cannot be used for disciplinary matters. This MUST be taken into account in the study design.

Multi-disciplinary and open discussion

An audit is more likely to be successful if it has the enthusiastic support of all the staff concerned. It will have implications for professions and disciplines other than your own, and so they should be consulted and involved at an early stage. The best way to achieve this is to form an audit group which incorporates representatives from all the teams involved in delivering the service. Involving patients in the process is also considered desirable.

Regular discussion sessions are an important part of audit; the project will benefit and in fact requires input from relevant staff at certain key points.

It is crucial to have a consensus meeting (i.e. a meeting in which all specialties and teams are represented) where agreement is reached that the topic is important (otherwise they are unlikely to help to develop and implement any changes) and on the standards against which you will assess health care (or else they may reject your findings on the grounds that they were inappropriate benchmarks).

For the same reason, another consensus meeting should be held once you have collected your data, so that you can agree that you have identified an important problem, and so you can think about how you are going to change the service and over what timescale you will implement this.

As a rule of thumb, people are far more receptive to change and willing to cooperate in something for which they are responsible than in something which is imposed from an external source.

The most important points of the cycle are summarized in Figure 10.4. It is worth remembering these for exams and interviews.

Types of audit

Audits can be categorized into the areas of care that they look at:

- Audits of structure:
  - What health-care facilities are there?
  - What buildings, equipment and staff are available?
  - Typically more of a management issue than a clinician's problem.
    e.g. Looking at staffing levels / bedspaces and how this impacts upon A&E trolley waits.
- Audits of process:
  - Did the patient receive the best possible care?
  - The most common type of audit
  - It considers the investigations, diagnosis and treatment given
  - Was the care done (or given) as it was originally intended to be?

e.g. did patients with an acute myocardial infarct receive thrombolysis within six hours?

- Audits of outcome:
  - What was the end result for the patient?
  - How successful was the intervention for the patient?
  - In other words, did the intervention have the expected benefit, or were there any adverse effects?
  - Perhaps the most difficult type of audit because the consequences can be varied and subtle. They can also be extremely subjective
  - Especially difficult when considering chronic processes
  - BUT it is the most relevant type of audit as it asks 'How did the patient do?'
    e.g. the national Confidential Enquiry into Maternal and Sudden Infant Deaths (implemented by NICE).

As discussed in Chapter 4, there are a number of different measures for patient outcomes. Death is the most extreme outcome; mortality figures are regularly audited for peri-operative care (a national audit set up and run by NICE). Other measures include morbidity (how disabled a person is after the intervention), QALYS (quality adjusted life years) and patient satisfaction. The difficulty of course with these is that there is a wide variation in how one interprets such 'soft' measures. They rely on subjective values of the doctor or the patient and frequently both.

Why audit doesn't always work

In an ideal world there would be no barriers to audit. However, there are both practical and political considerations:

- Set reasonable expectations – you cannot cure the NHS of all its woes overnight!
- Does everyone see it as important a topic as you do? Unless the audit findings are seen as a priority (by senior colleagues or other departments) no change will be effected. This highlights the need for a consensus of opinion and constant discussion.
- There may be different motives behind an audit. Managers may well request an audit because of political pressure on them – if so, the auditors' agenda will be quite different from the managers'.

For example:
- An A&E physician may want to perform an 'audit of process' in acute myocardial infarcts (e.g. how quickly they were triaged, investigated and definitive care given).
- The management may want to have an 'audit of structure' within the A&E (e.g. lack of bedspaces, staff shortages and the ensuing trolley waits meaning that the patient with a myocardial infarct was not taken to CCU).

- Audits can often run into problems when they do not consider this 'ideological mismatch' between the agendas of clinicians, managers and auditors.
- Be aware of other reasons why audit does not effect change – it may be a political rather than practical obstacle.

How to do your own audit

The government has earmarked specific resources for audit. Within each Trust there are Clinical Audit Departments that have staff specifically trained to advise and assist in any of the stages of an audit. They are your resource, and there to help you! Use them. Plan your audit carefully and remember that data collection (although the most obvious step) can only happen once you are clear exactly what information you are trying to find out:

1. Choose a topic.
2. Create an audit team (remember – in order to be effective it needs input from all the various disciplines involved in providing the service).
3. Hold a consensus meeting to:
   a. Agree on the importance of the topic.
   b. Set aims and objectives.
   c. Develop standards.
4. Select an audit sample.
5. Design a data collection form.
6. Pilot the audit.
7. COLLECT THE DATA!
8. Analyse the information and write the audit report.
9. Present your results and hold another consensus meeting.
10. Implement.
11. Publish your results.
12. Re-audit (after an appropriate length of time).

- Discuss the importance of understanding and learning how clinical audit works.
- Explain the basic principles of audit.
- Outline the different types of audit.
- Outline the steps involved in carrying out an audit.
- Describe the difficulties involved and the measures taken to tackle them in 'setting standards'.

References
Crombie IK, Davies HT 1993 Missing link in the audit cycle. Quality in Health Care 2(1): 47–8
Healy K 1998 Why clinical audit doesn't work. Success depends on type of audit. British Medical Journal 316(7148): 1906

Further reading
Chambers R, Boath E 2000 Clinical effectiveness and clinical governance made easy. 2nd edn. Oxford: Radcliffe Medical Press Ltd. pp. 1–63, 117–46
NHS Executive 1996 Promoting Clinical Effectiveness. London: NHS Executive

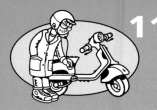

11. Critical Appraisal of Journals

Don't believe everything you read

The era of evidence-based medicine (EBM) has arrived. Naturally this has been received with mixed reactions in the medical community. EBM is the enhancement of a clinician's traditional skills in diagnosis, treatment, prevention and related areas through the systematic framing of relevant and answerable questions and the use of mathematical estimates of probability and risk.

It is vital for all medical professionals to critically appraise their current practice. Doctors need to keep up to date with their knowledge throughout their career, not only for the purpose of exams, but so that they can make patient care more objective, more customized, more logical and more cost-effective.

However, as with all things in medicine, caution must be exercised. Every month around 5000 medical journals are published worldwide and only 11–15% of the material in print today will subsequently prove to be of scientific value. Do not accept clinical evidence blindly. There are several databases for searching the plethora of literature. Medline, compiled by the National Library of Medicine, is the easiest. It is a good idea to book a session with a trained librarian to familiarize yourself with it.

According to Jones et al. (1995), there are three basic levels of reading the literature, as illustrated in Figure 11.1.

Journal clubs have been set up as part of most undergraduate medical courses, and are almost always present for practising doctors in various hospitals. They prove invaluable in gaining an insight into sequentially evaluating the current research on a particular topic. The more you practise appraising the evidence presented to you, the better you will become at quickly judging a poor study from a good one.

An approach to the appraisal of clinical papers and studies

Most papers found in medical journals have the following format:
- Introduction.
- Methods.
- Results.
- Discussion.

In order to decide the value of a paper, one must assess the design of the study and not just the value of the hypothesis. Remember that the results can be statistically significant, but if the methodology of the study is flawed, no great benefits to the patient can be accrued by implementing the findings.

A systematic approach to reading any paper is recommended as follows:
- *Identify the purpose of the study and assess the hypothesis that the authors are testing* – The introduction of any paper should adequately

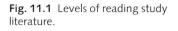
Fig. 11.1 Levels of reading study literature.

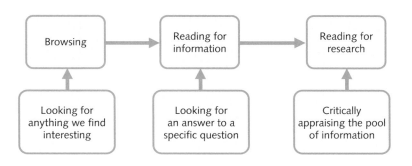

highlight these areas. It will also give an overview of the current research in the area and what prompted the authors to do their research. Another crucial point to remember is that most scientists seek to disprove the *null hypothesis* and instead try to show a difference between the various groups in their study. However, these days, both quantitative and qualitative research is seen as being more than just about hypothesis testing.

- *Evaluate the type of study design* – Primary studies report actually performed research. Secondary (integrative) studies summarize and draw conclusions from primary studies (Fig. 11.2). There are several terms that one must understand when reading clinical research studies (Fig. 11.3).
- *Decide whether the design of the study is appropriate for the research questions posed* – Most studies fall into the categories mentioned in Figure 11.4. Not all studies need to be randomized-controlled trials (RCTs).

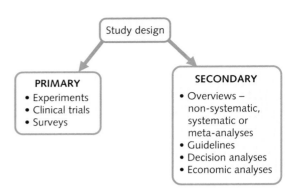

Fig. 11.2 Study design.

new piece of research you need to assess whether the findings of the study will add to the already existing literature. Also check if any similar studies have been conducted before.

Who is the study about?

Compare the patients used in the study to the ones you see on an everyday basis. There is no point in trying to adopt a new approach based on a study that kept patients in a state-of-the-art hospital with continuous 24-hour monitoring. Other aspects to pay attention to are:

- *The recruitment of subjects* – Placing an advertisement on the internet already opens the study to *recruitment bias* as you are selecting only computer-literate people. It might be better to recruit every 1 in 100 patients who walked into

Evaluating methodological quality

This is the most important aspect of any study. Spending time on this section will guide you in selecting the best evidence. You need to ask yourself several questions.

Was the study original?

A small proportion of medical research is on groundbreaking discoveries. Some studies aim to better an originally tested hypothesis, e.g. meta-analysis. For a

Fig. 11.3 Terms used in clinical studies.

Terms used in clinical studies	
Term	**Meaning**
Single-blinded	Only subjects do not know which treatment they are being given
Double-blinded	Neither subjects nor investigators know who is receiving which treatment
Cross-over	Each subject receives both the active treatment and the control in random order, often separated by a *wash-out* period of no treatment
Placebo-controlled	Control subjects receive a placebo which mimics the active treatment, but has no clinical effect
Factorial design	A study that permits one to assess the effects, both separately and combined, of more than one independent variable on a given outcome

Source: adapted from Greenhalgh T 2003 How to Read a Paper – The Basics of Evidence-based Medicine, 2nd edn, London: BMJ Books, p. 44

Fig. 11.4 Preferred study design for each study area.

Preferred study design for each study area	
Area being assessed	**Preferred study**
Therapy	Randomized-controlled trials
Diagnosis	Cross-sectional survey
Screening	Cross-sectional survey
Prognosis	Longitudinal cohort study
Causation	Cohort, case-controlled and case-reports (these need to be interpreted with caution)

Source: adapted from Greenhalgh T 2003 How to Read a Paper – The Basics of Evidence-based Medicine, 2nd edn, London: BMJ Books, pp. 39–55

the A&E department, for instance, depending on what you intend to survey.

- *Exclusion criteria* – Many trials in the UK exclude patients with coexisting illness, those who do not speak English, the illiterate or the non-articulate. However, daily clinical practice yields itself to treating patients from diverse backgrounds.
- *Inclusion criteria* – RCTs may only focus on a particular class of patients and their findings cannot always be generalised to the broader population. For example, a drug trialled on severely hypertensive patients in hospital may not be applicable to those with mild hypertension in the community.
- *'Real life circumstances'* – Some studies will use rare, high-tech equipment or place their patients in special wards. This clearly cannot be translated into daily clinical practice.

How sensible is the design of the study?

Carefully evaluate the specific interventions being considered and against what others they are being compared; e.g. if Eureka Drugs Inc. releases 'Wondermycin' which prolongs life, you will want to know that it actually does so. You will not accept the use of a *surrogate marker* such as the activity of an obscure enzyme 'Longetivitase' which the company reports is a reliable marker of how long a person will live.

Was systematic bias taken into account?

Systematic bias is anything that erroneously falsifies the conclusions. It occurs in both RCTs and non-RCTs. In RCTs, one needs to evaluate *selection, performance, exclusion, and detection biases*. In non-RCTs, baseline characteristics of the populations of all groups should be comparable. However, this may prove difficult in cohort studies, so this must be taken into account when analysing the data. In case-controlled studies, there is always an element of bias as the doctor decides when a patient actually becomes a 'case'.

Was the assessment blinded?

Ideally, both patients and investigators should be blinded to treatment, but this is not always possible, e.g. if one is administered a new form of insulin, and the blood glucose is abnormally high, one will measure the blood glucose again for assurance. This is *performance bias*.

What about the statistics?

Before a trial begins, researchers can work out how large a sample they need in order to demonstrate a truly important difference between the two groups. This is also known as the *power* of a study. The mean and standard deviation of the principal outcome variable will also need to be taken into account. Underpowered studies usually suffer from *type II* or β errors where the authors find it harder than they anticipated recruiting their subjects, so they wrongfully draw the conclusion that the treatment had no effect. *Type I* or α errors are quite common and state that there is a significant difference in the various groups of the study, when actually it is due to a sampling error. The *duration* of follow-up must be adequate (e.g. there is no point in assessing the efficacy of a slimming diet for two days). Also a note of the patients who dropped out from the study must be made and their reasons for doing so.

Interpreting the results

In most cases, one does not need to be able to perform the various statistical tests, but one must

179

know what they mean. Furthermore, several statistics packages are available to do all the number-crunching. The paper in question should use the correct statistical analysis methods based on the data collected. For example, it is wrong to use a chi-squared test to compare the content of alcohol in the blood of rugby players on Fridays and Saturdays. A paired t-test is more appropriate.

Applying the findings

Clinical practice will undoubtedly become busier and the time for reading the vast amounts of literature all the more valuable. Synthesizing the information and drawing up conclusions that you can use to improve the quality of care that the patient receives is an asset worth acquiring. However, it requires a lot of practice.

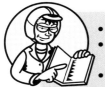

- Outline the role of journals in good medical practice.
- List the key areas that must be scrutinized in any paper before accepting the results of the study.
- Discuss what issues you would look at when assessing the methodology of a study.
- Describe how you would ensure that the results of a study are valid.
- Explain what factors would prompt you to draw sound inferences applicable to clinical practice, based on the results of a study.

Reference

Jones R, Knmonth A-L 1995 Critical Reading for Primary Care. Oxford: Oxford University Press

Further reading

Altman D 1991 Practical statistics for medical research. London: Chapman and Hall, pp. 461–2
Greenhalgh T 2003 How to Read a Paper – The Basics of Evidence-based Medicine, 2nd edn, London: BMJ Books, pp. 15–36, 39–55, 59–73

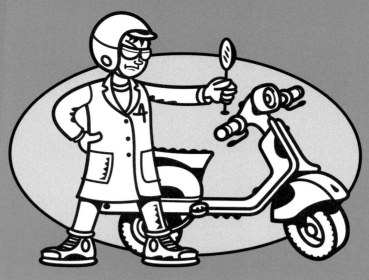

SELF-ASSESSMENT

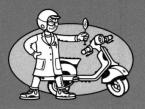

Indicate whether each answer is true or false.

1. National Screening programmes exist for:

(a) Phenylketonuria in male babies only.
(b) Cervical cancer screening for all women aged 20–64.
(c) HIV screening in all pregnant women.
(d) Abdominal aortic aneurysm.
(e) All women over 45 years, who undergo breast cancer screening.

2. Criteria for a new screening programme:

(a) A thorough understanding of the natural history of the disease.
(b) At the onset of the disease, a well-established effective treatment is available.
(c) A screening test with high specificity should be available.
(d) Resources are given to screen the whole population at once.
(e) A screening test with high sensitivity is needed.

3. Prevalence increases (all else being constant) with a:

(a) Growth in the size of the population.
(b) Rise in the incidence rate.
(c) Greater specificity in the diagnostic tests.
(d) Delayed recovery.
(e) Increase in survival time.

4. With regard to cohort studies:

(a) They cannot measure incidence.
(b) Subjects are selected as long as they have the condition whether under study or not.
(c) They are longitudinal in design.
(d) They are essential for estimating the prevalence of disease.
(e) To determine the frequency of the occurrence of the condition under study, subjects are studied over time.

5. With regard to case-control studies:

(a) The odds ratio is a good estimate of the disease incidence.
(b) There is prospective measurement of risk factors.
(c) They are not good for investigating rare diseases.
(d) For the risk factors under investigation, controls must be matched.
(e) The number of cases and controls must be equal.

6. Comparison of mortality rates in two different populations can be obtained by:

(a) Life expectancy at birth.
(b) Numbers of deaths in each group.
(c) Mean age at death.
(d) SMRs (standardised mortality ratios).
(e) Proportion of those aged above 80 years.

7. Disease notification:

(a) Provides reliable information about infectious diseases.
(b) Services are essential for health service planning.
(c) Services collect details of hospital bed usage.
(d) From claims of sickness benefit are unreliable.
(e) On cancer incidence is stored by cancer registries.

8. With regard to randomized-controlled trials:

(a) Patients are allocated randomly to treatments.
(b) The patients selected must be suitable for any of the arms of the study.
(c) Treatments are allocated randomly to patients.
(d) Observers of assessment are 'blinded' to who gets what treatment.
(e) The treatment is ineffective if there is a non-significant result in a trial.

9. In any given screening test:

(a) Falsely high prevalence rate results from low specificity.
(b) The percentage of truly negative subjects correctly classified by the test gives the specificity.
(c) High sensitivity means few false negatives.
(d) The higher the specificity, the lower the sensitivity.
(e) High repeatability guarantees high validity.

10. An epidemiological rate is regarded as crude if:

(a) It is based on an intercensal population estimate rather than a census figure.
(b) It covers five years rather than one.
(c) Its value is given per thousand instead of per hundred thousand.
(d) It is given only to two significant decimal figures.
(e) It fails to observe the benefit of separating different age groups.

11. A cross-sectional study differs from a cohort study in that:

(a) It is usually cheaper.
(b) Calculating relative risks is impossible.
(c) Incidence rates cannot be measured.
(d) It is not done on a defined population.
(e) Both disease and risk factors are ascertained at the same time.

12. **When using a sphygmomanometer to measure blood pressure:**

(a) Observers of the same sex as the subject produce higher readings.
(b) Repeated observations by the same observer will remove observer bias.
(c) Patients having extreme readings on one occasion are likely to be less extreme when the reading is repeated.
(d) Digit preference is a marker of the degree of imprecision.
(e) The normal blood pressure is 120/80 mmHg.

13. **Estimating the prevalence of a disease is possible using:**

(a) A survey of outpatients attending a general clinic.
(b) A cross-sectional survey.
(c) The percentage of hospital discharges with that diagnosis.
(d) Cases in a general practice with an age and sex register.
(e) The ratio of cases to controls in a case-controlled study.

14. **Vaccines:**

(a) Contribute towards 'herd' immunity.
(b) For MMR are used internationally.
(c) Can be effective after exposure to the infectious agent.
(d) Were largely responsible for the decline in mortality from infectious diseases in developed countries.
(e) Should be safer than therapies.

15. **Relative risk:**

(a) Is better than attributable risk for showing that a risk factor is likely to be causally associated with a disease.
(b) Quantifies the risk in absolute terms unlike the attributable risk.
(c) For a risk factor is usually the ratio of the risk of those with the factor and those without it.
(d) Can be estimated from a case-control study.
(e) Can be low for a factor with a high attributable risk.

16. **Trends in standardized mortality rates for a disease over time may be affected by:**

(a) Fashions in diagnosis.
(b) Acceptability of inadequate or vague diagnosis.
(c) The age and sex distribution of the population.
(d) Changes in medico-legal practice.
(e) Revision of the International Classification of Diseases.

17. **Epidemiological measures of disease frequency:**

(a) Mortality and case fatality rates are unequal.
(b) Unless rates are changing, the mortality rate cannot be greater than the incidence rate.
(c) If the incidence rate of a disease is increasing, there will be an increase in the case fatality rate.
(d) The incidence rate is reduced by an increase in the recovery rate.
(e) The prevalence rate will increase if average survival time decreases.

18. **In a case-control study:**

(a) Controls should be free of any known disease.
(b) The number of cases and controls must be equal.
(c) The case and control arms should have the same proportion of men to women.
(d) The history of exposure to risk factors should be obtained without knowledge of whether the subject is a case or a control.
(e) Cases and controls should be matched for all possible factors.

19. **In London a survey of car drivers killed in road accidents showed that half of them were wearing seat belts. It can be concluded that:**

(a) Only 50% of the car drivers were wearing seat belts.
(b) Seat belts decrease the risk of a fatality by half.
(c) Seat belts do not give complete protection from fatal injury.
(d) Not all car drivers wear seat belts.
(e) A control series of drivers who survive major accidents is needed.

20. **A valid comparison of mortality in different populations can be done using:**

(a) Indirectly age-standardized mortality rates.
(b) Age- and sex-specific mortality rates.
(c) Directly age-standardized mortality rates.
(d) Levels of life insurance claims.
(e) Mean age at death.

21. **Cigarette smoking is associated with an increase in mortality from cirrhosis of the liver, so:**

(a) Smoking should be stopped by patients with any evidence of liver disease.
(b) Tobacco smoke has a toxic effect on the liver.
(c) Cigarette smokers could have an increased incidence of cirrhosis or diminished survival in those with cirrhosis or both.
(d) In looking for evidence of causation it would be advisable to ensure that the heavy smoking led to the onset of the cirrhosis.
(e) Malignant secondary deposits in the liver are being misdiagnosed as cirrhosis.

22. **Examples of primary prevention include:**

(a) Self-examination of the breast for lumps.
(b) Measles, mumps and rubella (MMR) immunization.
(c) Smoking cessation after a myocardial infarction.
(d) Prevention of dental caries by fluoridation of water.
(e) Cervical cytology screening.

23. **A suitable screening test used to detect:**

(a) Early breast cancer is self-examination of the breasts.
(b) Diabetes is the glucose tolerance test.
(c) A disease should be cheap and acceptable.
(d) Phenylketonuria is routinely performed in the UK.
(e) Early disease should have a low coverage in those at risk.

24. **Epidemiology includes studying the:**

(a) Distribution and determinants of frequency of disease.
(b) Aetiology of disease.
(c) Frequency of causes of death.
(d) Patterns of financing and organization of health care.
(e) Determinants of frequency of disease.

25. **The relationship between low birth weight and intake of alcohol by the mother can be studied by taking detailed histories of the consumption of alcohol at the time of the prenatal visit. This type of study is a:**

(a) Correlation.
(b) Cross-section.
(c) Retrospective case-control.
(d) Clinical trial.
(e) Prospective-cohort.

26. **In a measure of central tendency:**

(a) The median is more sensitive than the mean to extreme observations.
(b) If more outlying observations are larger than the rest of the values, the median will be smaller than the mean.
(c) If more outlying observations are smaller than the rest of the values, the data are skewed to the right.
(d) For a symmetrical distribution, the mean and the median are equal, but the mode will be smaller than the mean.
(e) If the data are skewed to the right, the mean is larger than the median.

27. **Using the following denominators, we can calculate the rate of a disease:**

(a) Number of asymptomatic cases.
(b) Person-years of observation.
(c) Number of cases observed.
(d) Persons lost to follow-up.
(e) Number of new cases observed.

28. **Statistical inference:**

(a) A statistically significant test accepts the null hypothesis.
(b) A test of statistical significance does not prove causality.
(c) A confidence interval does not assess whether an association is due to bias.
(d) A confidence interval gives statistical significance as well as information concerning sample size.
(e) A statistically significant test suggests the small probability of a 'chance' occurrence.

29. **Randomization ensures that:**

(a) Placebo effects are eliminated.
(b) An equal number of subjects will be followed in the treatment and control group.
(c) Assignment of people to treatment and control groups occurs by chance.
(d) Treatment and control groups are alike in all respects except treatment.
(e) Bias in observations is eliminated.

30. **In comparing the difference between two mean blood pressure values, the value of P is 0.75, hence:**

(a) The difference occurred by chance.
(b) The difference is not statistically significant.
(c) The null hypothesis is rejected.
(d) Sampling variation is not a likely explanation of the difference.
(e) The difference is in line with the null hypothesis.

31. **Criteria for a public health surveillance system:**

(a) Evaluation of control and prevention measures.
(b) Evaluation of hypotheses about the occurrence of a disease.
(c) Detection of epidemics.
(d) Detection of rare but fatal conditions such as Alzheimer's disease.
(e) Description of the natural history and trends of a health condition.

32. **To calculate sample size, we need to know:**

(a) Magnitude of effect.
(b) Ratio of groups to be compared.
(c) Level of statistical significance, α error.
(d) The null hypothesis.
(e) Chance of missing a real effect, β error.

33. **A meta-analysis:**

(a) It is applied by collecting results of small, randomized controlled trials when no single trial has large enough numbers to reach statistical significance.
(b) Results are combined from different studies to obtain a numerical estimate of an overall effect.
(c) It is a study in which the units of analysis are populations or groups of people, rather than individuals.
(d) It is used to enhance the statistical power of research findings where numbers in available studies are too small.
(e) It is meant to be more objective and quantitative than a narrative review.

34. **Cohort studies:**

(a) Are essential to estimate the prevalence of disease.
(b) Subjects are observed over time to determine the frequency of occurrence of the condition under study.
(c) Are longitudinal in design.
(d) Can be retrospective.
(e) Subjects are selected on the basis of characteristics present before the onset of conditions being studied.

35. **Causality can be established by:**

(a) Consistency.
(b) Temporal sequence.
(c) Biological gradient.
(d) Strength of association.
(e) Concurrency.

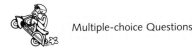
36. When testing a new medical treatment, suitable control groups include patients who are:

(a) Unwilling to receive the new treatment.
(b) Treated by a different doctor simultaneously.
(c) Not suitable for the new treatment.
(d) Treated in a different hospital.
(e) Ex-patients of the doctor conducting the study.

37. Placebos are essential in clinical trials:

(a) Because they may help to conceal the subject's treatment from assessors.
(b) Because the fact of being treated may itself produce a response.
(c) To guarantee comparability in non-randomized trials.
(d) When an active treatment is to be compared to no treatment.
(e) When two apparently similar active treatments are to be compared.

38. A population:

(a) May be infinite.
(b) May be any set of things that one wishes to study.
(c) May consist of things that do not actually exist.
(d) Consists only of people.
(e) May be finite.

39. Advantages of random sampling are that:

(a) The sample can be drawn from a 'known population'.
(b) It is easy to perform.
(c) It can be applied to any population.
(d) It is unbiased.
(e) Likely errors can be estimated.

40. Pulse pressure in women has a distribution that skews to the right. So:

(a) The majority of observations will be more than 1 standard deviation from the mean.
(b) About 95% of observations will be expected to be within 2 standard deviations of the mean.
(c) Fewer observations will be below the mean than above it.
(d) The standard deviation will estimate the accuracy of pulse pressure.
(e) The standard deviation will be approximately equal to the mean.

41. After treatment with Fantasticillin, 80% of patients are completely recovered:

(a) We need to know about the control group.
(b) The number of significant figures used suggests a degree of precision.
(c) This statement is misleading.
(d) There might be a very small number of patients.
(e) Fantasticillin is a great drug.

42. The following statistics are adjusted to allow for the age distribution of the population:

(a) Perinatal mortality rate.
(b) Crude mortality rate.
(c) Expectation of life at birth.
(d) Fertility rate.
(e) Standardized mortality rate.

43. If the size of a random sample is increased, we would expect that the:

(a) Degrees of freedom for the estimated variance would increase.
(b) Sample variance would increase.
(c) Standard error of the mean would decrease.
(d) Standard deviation would decrease.
(e) Mean would increase.

44. Shortcomings and weaknesses of the NHS include:

(a) Lack of receptiveness with a certain degree of lack of choice for patients.
(b) Lack of services with many user charges.
(c) Restricted access to latest technology.
(d) Incompetent staff because of a lack of high-quality training.
(e) Interference by ministers in the fine details of health-care management.

45. Desirable outcomes of a successful disease-prevention programme are:

(a) To offer the greatest benefit to the largest number of people.
(b) The targeting of high-risk individuals which will decrease the overall burden of disease.
(c) A population-based approach with a smaller benefit in a larger number of individuals which will yield better results.
(d) The need to identify a high-risk group.
(e) To reduce the damage the disease causes.

46. Ethics of screening:

(a) A false positive result can cause unnecessary anxiety.
(b) There may not be any other unplanned effects of a positive test.
(c) A false negative result will give false reassurance.
(d) For the individual the screening test can do no harm and confer only benefit.
(e) There may be a risk attached to the screening test or subsequent diagnostic test.

47. Statistical terms used in medicine:

(a) A random sample is one in which any individual or unit has an equal chance of being represented.
(b) A population always relates to a geographical group of individuals.
(c) The frequency is the number of times a particular event occurs in a population.
(d) Terms like variance, standard deviation and range are essential for manipulating the data to interpret useful conclusions.
(e) A collection of items of information is a data set.

48. Evidence-based medicine:

(a) Can provide ways for formulating a coordinated plan for the management of disease by a multi-disciplinary team.
(b) Provides no allowance to improve the quality and efficiency of disease-management procedures.
(c) Identifies gaps in the current state of knowledge and highlights areas requiring more investigation.
(d) Provides a robust way of managing disease but does not enhance the clinical outcome.
(e) Does not provide a way for synthesizing the vast amounts of information from medical literature.

49. A clinical audit does not always work because:

(a) Expectations set are unreasonable.
(b) The audit findings are not seen as a priority by senior colleagues and other departments and change will be effected.
(c) There may be excessive political interference.
(d) There is 'ideological mismatch' among clinicians', managers' and auditors' agendas.
(e) The managers and the auditors have different reasons for carrying it out.

50. Analysing research papers in medical journals:

(a) The recruitment of subjects should be devoid of recruitment bias.
(b) Carefully interpret the exclusion criteria and subsequent findings.
(c) Benefit shown by using a novel, high-tech robot to operate can be replicated in a normal routine operating theatre.
(d) Only accept the findings if the study was carried out as a randomized-controlled trial.
(e) Ignore the inclusion criteria.

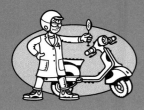

Short-answer Questions (SAQs)

Ethics

1. What is utilitarianism? What are its strengths and weaknesses?

2. What is Kantianism? What are its strengths and weaknesses?

3. What is 'virtue ethics'? What are its strengths and weaknesses?

4. What are the 'four principles'? And what does each one mean?

5. What is a moral right?

6. Describe the necessary steps for a case of medical negligence to succeed in the UK courts.

7. Your patient has cancer, your patient's son asks you not to reveal the diagnosis. What ethical principles should you consider?

8. Describe how you can obtain valid consent.

9. Describe the circumstances in which confidentiality should not be maintained and why?

10. Explain the ageist accusation against the use of QALYs.

11. Describe the pro-life and pro-choice positions in the abortion debate.

12. Describe the positions for and against active euthanasia.

13. Organ markets are morally acceptable. Discuss.

Sociology

14. How do symptoms affect the behaviour of those who fall ill?

15. Why would people choose to visit a practitioner of alternative medicine?

16. What is stigma? How does it differ from labelling?

17. How would you characterize a paternalistic doctor–patient relationship?

18. What is 'patient-centredness'?

19. With reference to hospital admission, what is depersonalization? And why does it occur?

20. How is a patient's self-identity affected in chronic illness?

21. Outline the differences between impairment, disability and handicap.

22. What are the typical stages of dying (as described by Kubler-Ross)?

23. What is the 'materialist' explanation for health inequalities?

24. What sort of social causes are there for health inequalities between men and women?

25. How can social structures be seen to create dependency in elderly people?

Statistics

26. One thousand adults in Sheffield are screened for carcinoma of the colon. Three hundred and thirty have a positive screening result. These people are then offered a gold standard diagnostic test for this malignancy and all accept it. Forty-five of them are found to have carcinoma of the colon on administration of the diagnostic test. The original 1000 people are followed up for two years and five people who tested negative on the screening test develop the disease, which is confirmed by the diagnostic test. Fill in the two-by-two table below:

	People who have disease confirmed by 'gold standard'	People who DO NOT have disease confirmed by 'gold standard'	
Positive screening test			
Negative screening test			
TOTAL			Total population

   (a) What is the prevalence of the disease in this population?
   (b) What is the predictive value of a positive screening test in this population?
   (c) What is the predictive value of a negative screening test in this population?
   (d) What is the sensitivity of the screening test?
   (e) What is the specificity of the screening test?

27. Since you are a keen medical student, Dr Jones has asked you to determine the amount of diabetes currently in his general practice population. What type of study design is most appropriate to do this? What are the epidemiological problems you would encounter and how would you control them?

28. As part of reducing health inequalities and tackling social exclusion, the government is keen to reduce unwanted teenage pregnancies. Outline a strategy for achieving this in an inner-city area. What sources of data would you use to evaluate progress with your strategy?

29. From your clinical experience you develop a hypothesis that there is a direct association between the amount of beer drunk and myocardial infarction. You decide to test this by obtaining statistics on the average consumption of beer in each of several countries in Europe and comparing these with published death rates from myocardial infarction for each of these countries:

   (a) What type of study is this?
   (b) What are the advantages and disadvantages of this type of study?

30. Define the following terms:
   (a) Incidence
   (b) Prevalence
   (c) Attributable risk.

31. Randomization is considered to make the RCT study design 'superior' to other analytical studies such as case-control or cohort studies. Why? What do you understand by the intention to treat analysis?

32. You have been asked to investigate an outbreak of salmonellosis at the annual dinner held at the Royal College of Physicians. Outline the preliminary steps you would take.

33. Compare and contrast the following terms: mean, mode and median.

34. Outline the reasons for practising evidence-based medicine and some of the problems regularly encountered with its practice.

35. List the key features of a clinical audit.

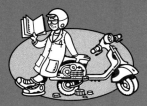

Essay Questions

1. What is medical ethics?

2. Compare and contrast the three major schools of ethical thought.

3. Outline the strengths and weaknesses of the 'four principles' approach to medical ethics.

4. Is lying to a patient ever morally permissible?

5. What are the components of informed consent?

6. When is the disclosure of confidential information morally justifiable?

7. What are the necessary conditions for conducting a research trial?

8. Describe the various methods of resource allocation.

9. Cloning human beings is never justifiable. Discuss.

10. Involuntary treatment is always morally unjustifiable. Discuss.

11. Describe some of the reasons for the increasing popularity of alternative medicine.

12. What is normality?

13. How has the doctor–patient relationship changed over the past century?

14. Compare and contrast the paternalistic, consumerist, mutual and default doctor–patient relationships.

15. Explain how conflict within the doctor–patient relationship can be minimized.

16. Explain the difference between compliance and concordance.

17. What social problems are experienced by the chronically ill?

18. How is the government trying to reduce inequality between the social classes?

19. Describe the inequalities in health between ethnic groups and discuss the differing explanations for such inequalities.

20. Describe the medical and social problems that are particular to the elderly.

21. Describe the evolution of the NHS since its birth in the 1940s to the present day.

22. Discuss the advantages and disadvantages of different health-care systems.

23. Outline the WHO criteria for any screening programme and highlight the ethical arguments associated with screening.

24. Identify the various areas that must be looked at when evaluating a statistical association.

25. Compare and contrast the different types of studies used in epidemiology.

26. Highlight the factors that could result in poor uptake of vaccination.

27. List the sources of routine data and argue the case for and against their use in epidemiology.

28. Briefly outline the stages of pharmacological research and development.

29. Identify the key steps in performing a clinical audit.

30. Explain the different health-care strategies you would use to decrease the mortality and morbidity associated with diabetes mellitus in your local town.

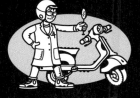

MCQ Answers

1. (a) False. All babies
   (b) True – but do those most at risk accept screening?
   (c) True – being introduced right now
   (d) False
   (e) False – The age range is 45–64, optional for those over 64 and no routine check-up for them

2. (a) True
   (b) True
   (c) False – for detecting all cases, high sensitivity is very important
   (d) False – repeated screening vital
   (e) True

3. (a) False – population growth will not affect it as the prevalence includes the denominator
   (b) True
   (c) False – due to fewer false positives, the reported prevalence will decline
   (d) True – prevalence increases if there is improved survival or slower recovery or cure rates in a given population
   (e) True

4. (a) False – unlike case-control studies, they can measure incidence
   (b) False – subjects are included for being part of a population or following an exposure
   (c) True
   (d) False
   (e) True

5. (a) False – the odds ratio gives a good estimate of relative risk
   (b) False – in people who are already affected by the disease (cases) and those who are not (controls), the risk factors/exposures are measured retrospectively
   (c) False – excellent for rare diseases
   (d) False – we obtain controls to check how common the risk is in people not already affected by the disease, so we do not match for the risk factor, e.g. smoking
   (e) False – often there are more controls

6. (a) True – using the death risks at different ages, we can calculate life expectancy at birth
   (b) False – the number at risk, the time span and the death risk will determine the number of deaths per group
   (c) False – the proportion of people at different ages will affect this
   (d) True – standardization means that differences in the age structure of the population have been accounted for
   (e) False – birth rate and migration are not taken into account

7. (a) True
   (b) True
   (c) True
   (d) True – not reliable and disease must have lasted more than seven days
   (e) True

8. (a) True – either the patients are randomly allocated to the treatment or vice-versa and the result is the same
   (b) True
   (c) True
   (d) False – there is no mention of double-blind in the question
   (e) False – sample size may be too small and power may be too low, but effect may be seen in a larger trial

9. (a) True – low specificity means a greater proportion of false positives thus high prevalence rate
   (b) True
   (c) True
   (d) True
   (e) False – a test must be repeatable if it is valid but not necessarily the other way round

10. (a) False – rates are usually based on mid-year populations
    (b) False
    (c) False – it can be any denominator
    (d) False
    (e) True – hence crude

11. (a) True
    (b) False
    (c) True – incidence can be measured only over time and not at one point in time
    (d) False – for both a denominator or defined population is vital
    (e) True – in a cross-sectional study, prevalence of disease is identified during the same time in the survey as the risk factors

12. (a) False
    (b) False – even though it may lower the effect of random variation in the reading, there will still be systematic bias
    (c) True – this phenomenon is called regression to the mean and occurs with unstable factors such as blood pressure
    (d) True – clinicians tend to round off readings to 0s and 5s
    (e) False – blood pressure is widely distributed, so a range exists

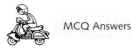

13. (a) False – a biased sample of the population
    (b) True
    (c) False – hospital inpatients are a biased sample of the population
    (d) True – but would only give the prevalence rate within that practice
    (e) False – usually determined by the investigator and is usually a simple multiple, e.g. in a case-control study the prevalence of a rare disease may be 1/1 000 000

14. (a) True
    (b) True
    (c) True – vaccines can be effective post-exposure in diseases, e.g. rabies
    (d) False – the major decline in mortality started before the introduction of vaccines and was probably due to improved nutritional and socio-economic status
    (e) True – since they are given to healthy individuals, the safety standards should be high

15. (a) True – the higher the relative risk, the more likely the association is to be causal
    (b) False – attributable risk is the risk difference rather than the risk ratio
    (c) True
    (d) True – case-control studies are widely used to estimate the relative risk
    (e) True – the relative risk for death from coronary disease in a heavy smoker is twice that in a non-smoker and the attributable risk is very high; for lung cancer the relative risk is 30 times but the attributable risk is lower

16. (a) True
    (b) True
    (c) False – age and sex standardization of mortality rates overcomes differences in these factors and enables valid comparisons to be made
    (d) True – only if you are actively seeking the condition will you ascribe it
    (e) True

17. (a) True – as mortality rate refers to death rate from the disease in a defined population, while the fatality rate is that among cases of the disease
    (b) True – if all new cases die, mortality rate is equal to the incidence rate
    (c) False – the proportion of cases that end in fatalities over a defined time period is likely to be independent of the incidence rate
    (d) False – the rate at which new cases appear in those previously unaffected will not be affected by what happens to cases subsequently
    (e) False – the proportion of the population with the disease will be increased by improved survival or by slower recovery or cure rates

18. (a) False – patients may be suffering from other diseases not being measured
    (b) False – most of the time this is the case, especially when cases and controls have been pair-matched, but if the number of cases is small, it is better to have more controls
    (c) False – the sex of the patients does not matter provided that the disease is not specific to a particular sex
    (d) True – there is investigator bias in the ascertainment of risk-factor exposure between cases and controls
    (e) False – if you match for a factor, you cannot investigate its contribution as a risk factor

19. (a) False – we do not know the prevalence of belt wearing either in survivors or motorists generally
    (b) False – this would only be true if wearing had no effect on survival
    (c) True – or no-one who died would be wearing one
    (d) True – if all drivers wore belts, all drivers killed would be wearing belts
    (e) True – this would show the degree of benefit of wearing a belt for those involved in a major accident

20. (a) True – indirect age standardization results in the commonly used indicator of comparative mortality known as the standardized mortality ratio
    (b) True – this is the purpose of these rates
    (c) True
    (d) False – majority of the population does not take out life insurance, some individuals take out several policies and a large proportion of policies elapse
    (e) False – mean age at death is likely to be affected greatly by the age structure of the population, patterns of fertility and migration, which will distort the effect of mortality rates alone

21. (a) False – people should stop smoking but based on the above evidence the association in itself is too weak to imply that cessation of smoking will improve the prognosis of cirrhosis
    (b) False – association does not always imply causation
    (c) True – increased mortality with one or both of the above mechanisms
    (d) True – it is crucial to check whether an association might be an effect of the disease and not a cause
    (e) False – this is a possible explanation, it does not follow from the observed association

22. (a) False – it does not prevent breast cancer but only facilitates in finding existing disease early
    (b) True – to prevent infection in healthy children
    (c) False – prevention of recurrences is secondary prevention
    (d) True – fluoride is incorporated into teeth and primarily prevents occurrence of caries
    (e) False – cervical smears are examined for early evidence of disease and prevention of progression to severe disease is known as secondary prevention

23. (a) True – easy to pick up breast lumps
    (b) False – although it is a useful diagnostic tool, but too time-consuming to perform
    (c) True
    (d) True – tested in neonates
    (e) False – however, it is often the case that those at greatest risk are the hardest to screen

24. (a) True – standard definition
    (b) False
    (c) False – it does not deal with mortality alone
    (d) False – this tne eventual aim of translating epidemiology into patient benefit
    (e) False

25. (a) False – not a type of study
    (b) False – not just a proportion of mothers visiting the clinic are being studied, all need to be included
    (c) False – we are not scrutinizing old records to determine the subjects, but vice versa
    (d) False – there is no control arm to the study
    (e) True – the subjects are categorized on the basis of exposure to the risk factor (alcohol intake) and then followed up to determine the outcome (low birth-weight)

26. (a) False – more robust and less sensitive to extreme observations
    (b) True – also the data are skewed to the right
    (c) False – to the left
    (d) False – the mean, mode and median are all the same for a symmetrical distribution
    (e) True

27. (a) False – patients may have the disease but are asymptomatic at that point in time
    (b) True – allows for variable follow-up periods, takes into account the number of subjects under observation and the duration of observation of each person
    (c) False – does not allow for standardization of follow-up periods
    (d) False – not related to the disease
    (e) False – eliminates those patients who already have the disease

28. (a) False – it rejects the null hypothesis
    (b) True
    (c) True
    (d) True
    (e) True

29. (a) False – a placebo might be the second arm of the study
    (b) False – highly unlikely
    (c) True
    (d) False – there will always be some chance differences, but provided that these are small, it is all right
    (e) False – some form of bias always exists

30. (a) False – only true if the null hypothesis is correct
    (b) True – statistical significance achieved if $P<0.05$
    (c) False – it is accepted
    (d) False – possible contribution to the difference
    (e) True

31. (a) True
    (b) True
    (c) True
    (d) False – detection of fatal conditions that have no treatment or improved prognosis from early detection and intervention is not an effective use of resources
    (e) True

32. (a) True
    (b) True
    (c) True
    (d) False – it is the main objective of the study, so cannot be used to calculate the sample size
    (e) True

33. (a) True
    (b) True
    (c) False – meta-analyses combine data from several studies, ecological studies use data based on groups of people as opposed to individuals
    (d) True
    (e) True

34. (a) False – estimated from cross-sectional studies
    (b) True
    (c) True – group of subjects defined and followed over time (prospective) or if cohort identified from past records (retrospective)
    (d) True
    (e) True

35. (a) True
    (b) True
    (c) True
    (d) True
    (e) False – even if the cause and effect occurred at the same time, such as in a cross-sectional survey, there is no proof of causality; the cause must precede the effect in time

36. (a) False
    (b) False – controls should be treated in the same place at the same time, under the same conditions
    (c) False – all patients should be willing to receive either treatment
    (d) False
    (e) False

37. (a) True
    (b) True
    (c) False – only in RCTs can we make a comparison between the different treatments
    (d) True
    (e) False – purpose of a placebo is to make dissimilar treatments appear similar

38. (a) True
    (b) True
    (c) True
    (d) False – a population can constitute anything
    (e) True

39. (a) True
    (b) False – some populations are very difficult to list
    (c) False – some populations cannot be identified
    (d) True
    (e) True

40. (a) False – within 1 standard deviation
    (b) True
    (c) False – more observations will be below the mean than above; median<mean
    (d) False – standard deviation measures the spread across people, not in one individual, which is vital for accuracy
    (e) False

41. (a) True
    (b) True
    (c) True – the denominator is not given and there is no control group for comparison
    (d) True – we may only have five patients of whom four got better
    (e) False – inconclusive information

42. (a) False
    (b) False
    (c) True – expectation of life does not depend on age distribution
    (d) False
    (e) True

43. (a) True – degrees of freedom = $n - 1$
    (b) False – it should neither increase nor decrease
    (c) True
    (d) False – it should neither increase nor decrease
    (e) False – it should neither increase nor decrease

44. (a) True
    (b) False – many services with few user charges
    (c) True
    (d) False
    (e) True

45. (a) True
    (b) False – it will benefit only this group
    (c) True – the aim is to eradicate, eliminate or minimize the impact of disease
    (d) False – the strategy targets all
    (e) True – a modifiable risk factor: cessation of smoking can retard progression of disease, e.g. lung cancer

46. (a) True – a screening test is a medical intervention done to a person who is not ill
    (b) False – e.g. a positive HIV result may alter your insurance premium
    (c) True
    (d) False – can be both harmful and beneficial
    (e) True

47. (a) True
    (b) False – it is the collection of all possible values of a given variable, e.g. patient records in a GP practice can be the population
    (c) False
    (d) True
    (e) True

48. (a) True
    (b) False – it allows for the above
    (c) True
    (d) False – evidence-based medicine provides a way for both managing the disease and enhancing the clinical outcome
    (e) False – its purpose is to evaluate the pool of medical literature and translate the findings into patient benefit

49. (a) True – expectations should be reasonable and practical
    (b) True – if it is not seen as a priority and there is no consensus of opinion nor constant discussion, the clinical audit will not work
    (c) True
    (d) False – the audit runs into problems if there is a mismatch
    (e) True

50. (a) True – recruitment bias prevents effective randomization without which the validity of the study decreases
    (b) True
    (c) False – without the expensive equipment, you cannot use the findings of the paper to benefit your patients
    (d) False – some questions cannot be assessed by using randomized controlled trials, e.g. whether mobile phones cause brain cancer
    (e) False – you cannot confidently state that coronary artery bypass surgery is better than angioplasty in the elderly if the research papers you looked at studied only those under the age of 50 years

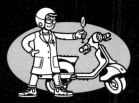

SAQ Answers

Ethics

1. Utilitarianism is a form of consequentialism. This means that it emphasizes the importance of 'good' consequences over other moral concerns such as rights and duties. Utilitarianism was founded by Jeremy Bentham and John Stuart Mill who defined 'utility' in terms of pleasure or happiness. Utilitarianism can be summed up as the 'greatest good for the greatest number' because it argues that the 'good' or right act is that which produces the greatest well-being. The strengths of utilitarianism include the fact that it incorporates a principle of equality – valuing the happiness of each person equally, and that it is based on a single principle of maximizing utility. However, utilitarian theorising can lead to intuitively difficult problems – such as letting one person die to save many people and other examples of overriding the rights of a minority to produce pleasure for a majority. Furthermore, in practice, utilitarianism can place high moral burdens on individuals – by demanding heroic and saintly acts.

2. Kantianism is a form of deontology. This means that it emphasizes rules and duties rather than consequences. Kantianism takes its name from Immanuel Kant, who argued that morality was something that humans imposed upon themselves on account of being rational. Kant argued that reason alone could enable humans to ascertain what was morally right and wrong. Kant formulated the 'categorical imperative' in order to apply a consistent test for moral correctness to actions. There are three formulations of the categorical imperative. The first is a universalizability test – we can only act in a way that is consistent with everyone acting in the same way. The second emphasizes the equality of all rational beings, and the third entreats us to act as in a 'kingdom of ends' – that is an ideal society, where everyone else also perfectly obeys the moral law. The strengths of Kantianism are that its structure is quite clear, and that responsibility for actions is placed upon the individual. However, Kantianism is rather absolutist and may struggle to deal with complex real-life dilemmas.

3. Virtue ethics is a type of narrative ethics. This means that it emphasizes interpretation and context rather than abstract principle and rules. Reasoning is by analogy rather than deduction. Virtue ethics is rooted in Aristotlean thought. It advocates that the 'right' action is the sort of action that would be carried out by the 'virtuous individual'. Virtue is a function of character which can be cultivated. Its strengths include a more personal, readily identifiable moral theory that is flexible to individual scenarios. However, its inflexibility can be unhelpful when trying to compare one virtue against another, or even deciding whether one act can be considered virtuous or not.

4.
- Autonomy – or more correctly 'respect for autonomy' is the principle of respecting the decisions made by those capable of making decisions. Autonomy is more than simply doing what one wants. A person has to be able to reason and think about the potential choice, decide and then act on that decision, in order to be considered autonomous.
- Beneficence – the principle of providing benefits.
- Non-maleficence – the principle of avoiding doing harm.
- Justice – the principle of ensuring fairness and equity in the distribution of risks and benefits.

5. Moral rights can be considered to be 'insistent normative demands' that can be used to trump other moral concerns. This means rights are the sorts of things that can be used against other moral arguments in order to protect the interest of some group – usually a minority or defenceless group – from the will of the majority or a powerful group.

6. A case of medical negligence needs the plaintiff to establish that the defendant owed him a duty of care and that the care provided failed to reach a reasonable standard of care, and that this failure was the cause of the injury to the plaintiff for which they are seeking damages.

7. There is a conflict of autonomy and beneficence in this scenario. The common (Western) opinion is that autonomy would overrule beneficence in this case – not revealing a diagnosis to a patient is considered *paternalistic*.

8. Consent for a procedure normally has to be obtained by someone who is able to do the procedure proposed. Details about the diagnosis and prognosis with and without treatment should be given. Benefits and probabilities of successful treatment as well as uncertainties, potential side effects and complications of a treatment should be explained. If alternatives exist, the details of these should also be explained. The patient should be reminded that they can change their mind at any time, and that they have the right to a second opinion. If students may be present at the procedure or if the procedure could be carried out by someone in training, the patient should be informed of this.

9. There are a number of occasions when confidential information can be disclosed. These include: with the patient's consent, within teams, in the patient's best interest, in the interest of others (to avoid serious harm or death), or if the disclosure is required by statute or the courts.

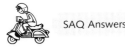

10. This accusation claims that the use of QALYs in deciding the allocation of resources is unfair. The argument runs that QALYs are inherently ageist because they prioritize the treatment of those with the greatest number of possible life years.

11. The pro-life position holds that life is sacrosanct, and that abortion is the equivalent of killing innocent life. Fetuses are seen as being morally equivalent to other humans or being potential human beings which also require moral protection. The pro-choice position identifies the pregnant woman as of primary importance – claiming that her choice to carry the pregnancy or not overrules any rights the fetus may or may not have. It often assumes that the fetus is not a *person* in the same way that the mother is – however, some authors have claimed that even if the fetus was the sort of entity considered to be a *person,* abortion would still be justifiable, given the dependency on the pregnant woman and the possible deleterious consequences for her.

12. Arguments in favour of active euthanasia can be based on consistency – we accept suicide, passive euthanasia and the doctrine of double effect – and through an appeal to principles – particularly autonomy or beneficence. Arguments against active euthanasia include the idea that it is unnecessary – due to improvements in palliative care – that it may lead to exploitation or a slippery slope where depressed individuals, rather than just the terminally ill, are requesting euthanasia – and that it is against commonly held goals of medicine.

13. There is a need for more organs to be procured at the moment – as currently there is a shortfall of organs. However, there are many systems that may lead to an increase in organ supply – these include mandated choice, opt-out systems and organ markets. A utilitarian argument might support organ markets if they are more effective than other systems. The considerations that weigh against an organ market include arguments relating to human dignity and exploitation.

Sociology

14. Many factors affect the behaviour of those who fall ill. Mechanic (1978) noted the following with regard to signs and symptoms: their obviousness, perceived seriousness, the degree to which they disrupted normal life, their frequency or persistence and the tolerance of the individual towards their symptoms.

15. The commonly cited benefits of alternative medicine are the increased time and continuity available, the attention to the individual, the increased patient involvement, lay interpretation of illness, physical contact and the addressing of spiritual concerns.

16. Stigma and labelling both involve a negative evaluation about a condition; however, labelling is the process whereby individual characteristics are identified by others (such as the medical profession) as abnormal or a 'disease'. Stigma refers to the negative connotations surrounding an illness or disease label within wider society.

17. The Parsons model epitomizes the paternalistic doctor–patient relationship. The doctor has a high level of control within the consultation – dictating the goals and agenda, assuming that the patient has a similar agenda. The doctor acts beneficently towards the patient, but without due regard for patient autonomy.

18. The idea of patient-centredness is to remind us of the central position of the patient within the doctor–patient relationship. It emphasizes a mutual relationship that considers the biopsychosocial aspects of the patient consulting, the individual personalities of both the doctor and the patient, and an idea of shared responsibility and power within the consultation.

19. Depersonalization refers to a loss of self-identity that arises on admission to hospital. This occurs due to a combination of the patient losing their normal social roles, being treated as part of a group rather than as an individual, the impersonal nature of medical procedures, an institutionalized schedule and a lack of privacy.

20. Chronic illness can radically re-shape a person's conception of oneself. The term 'biographical disruption' has been used to describe this rethinking of one's biography and self-concept. 'Narrative reconstruction' describes the way in which coherence and stability is reintroduced to the new concept of being a person with a chronic disease.

21. Impairment is the loss or abnormality of psychological, physiological or anatomical structure or function. Disability is an inability to perform an activity which is considered normal for a human being. Handicap is the disadvantage that results from an impairment or disability.

22. The five stages of dying are denial, anger, bargaining, depression and acceptance.

23. The materialist explanation isolates deprivation of material goods as the cause of health inequalities between groups. There is an additive effect of deprivation – lack of money for food may lead to poor nutrition, which may lead to chronic illness in childhood, poor educational attainment, continued poor housing in adulthood, poor employment prospects, increased exposure to detrimental environments, and so on.

24. Social causes may be 'materialistic' or 'behavioural'. Materialistic explanations include the fact that women are more likely to experience poverty than men and, therefore, suffer increased morbidity. Behavioural explanations include the difference in drinking and cigarette smoking between the sexes.

25. Forced retirement at a given age is one social structure that in effect creates dependency in elderly people. As does the tendency to place elderly people in nursing or residential homes away from the gaze of the working section of the population.

Statistics

26.

	People who have disease confirmed by 'gold standard'	People who DO NOT have disease confirmed by 'gold standard'	
Positive screening test	45	285	330
Negative screening test	5	665	670
TOTAL	50	950	Total population 1000

(a) Number of people who have the disease divided by total population 50/1000 have the disease = 5%
(b) Number who have a positive screening test and have the disease divided by total number who had positive screening test = 45/330 = 13.6%
(c) Number who have a negative screening test and who do not have the disease divided by total number who had a negative screening test = 665/670 = 99%
(d) Number who screen positive and have the disease divided by total number who have the disease = 45/50 = 90%
(e) Number of people who have a negative screening test and who do not have the disease divided by all those who do not have the disease = 665/950 = 70%

27. Your aim is to estimate prevalence, hence a cross-sectional study design is most appropriate. The problems encountered are:
(a) Case definition: Is there an agreed case definition/criteria for how to define DM?
(b) Sample size: Is there a large enough sample? The bigger the sample, the smaller the confidence interval, i.e. the more likely it is that your findings will be truly representative of the whole population.
(c) Selection bias: If you only measure people who visit the practice, how representative are they of the overall population registered with you? May want to randomly select cases and invite to attend for a health check, but some will refuse this, so then you

have to ask if the non-responders are likely to be different from those who take up the offer of attending.
(d) Measurement bias: How will you measure the presence of DM? Blood glucose – fasting or random? Glucose tolerance test? Urinalysis? Self reporting? Need to decide on valid reliable simple test, and standardize approach for all patients. Also, ideally should use same laboratory for all test results.
(e) The age of the practice population may affect prevalence. It is wise to think about standardization or use of age-specific rates. Also remember the ethnic diversity of the practice, e.g. South Asians predominantly will cause inflation of the prevalence as this group has a genetic predisposition to the disease.

28. The UK has the worst rate of teenage pregnancy (under 16 year-olds) in Western Europe. Teenage pregnancy is associated with poorer outcomes for both mother and baby.
• Start with local needs assessment to:
  – Quantify the issue locally
  – Identify effective interventions
  – Identify current service provision and gaps in services.
• Approaches to reducing teenage pregnancy include the following:
  – Health education – sex education in schools. Seems to be effective, especially if linked to skills-building and practical information on where to go to obtain contraceptives. Peer-led approaches to school-based education currently being evaluated in the UK
  – Clinical interventions to prevent pregnancy – access to clinical services important. Family planning clinics, or other clinics, open at times when young people are likely to be able to attend? Access to emergency contraception?
• Need to link services with knowledge/sex education.
• Other possible interventions:
  – Tackling inequalities/community development approaches. Good general education seems to be associated with deferring pregnancy. You may want to look at community development approaches/ways of reducing poverty locally, providing educational opportunities, etc.
  – For those who are pregnant and go on to deliver, they will probably benefit from targeted support from, e.g. health visitors and social workers. Targeted antenatal care programmes may also contribute to better outcomes.
• Evaluate progress: Monitor local age-specific birth rates (available from ONS – Office of National Statistics) over time. Could also look at other sources e.g.:
  – Termination rates locally
  – Attendances at family planning or other relevant clinics
  – Attendance at school-based programmes
  – Social services/health visitor case load.

29.
   (a) Ecological: The unit of analysis is the population and not the individual. It is also descriptive (not analytic) and observational (not interventional).
   (b) Advantages are that it is cheap and quick, looks at broad associations to provide clues about causation. Disadvantages include the ecological fallacy (those who get the disease may not be those who consume the beer), and inability to assess confounding in individuals.

30.
   (a) Incidence: Quantifies the number of *new cases* of a disease within a specified time interval. Incidence measures events (a change from a healthy state to a diseased state), usually expressed as a proportion or rate.
   (b) Prevalence: The frequency of a disease in a population at a point in time. Prevalence is a proportion. It is the only measure of disease occurrence that can be obtained from cross-sectional studies. It measures the burden of disease in a population. Prevalence measures status (a condition: a subject affected by a specific disease).
   (c) Attributable risk is the **difference** between incidence in two groups, where one group is exposed to certain risk factors and the other is not.

31. The strength of randomization is that both known and unknown confounders are likely to be distributed equally among the groups. If done properly, this should minimize bias and result in comparable groups.
   • Intention to treat analysis: All eligible patients regardless of compliance with the protocol should be included in the analysis as this provides a more valid assessment of treatment efficacy as it relates to clinical practice. Also, if you analyse only the compliant patients, you are probably analysing a subset who differ from the rest of the trial population, so you are introducing selection bias into your analysis.

32. Identify the at-risk population, i.e. all those who attended the function. Ideally, they would be identified from a convenient register (e.g. guest lists and staffing rosters) but frequently asking attendees to identify other attendees may be required ('snowballing'). Initiate a type of analytical study, e.g. a retrospective cohort study would be usual. Come up with a plausible hypothesis to test. There also has to be adequate identification of at-risk population and adequate ascertainment of plausible exposures (particularly the different foods available). Questionnaires will have to be administered and should include identification of the subject (name, address, phone), susceptibility factors (age, sex, intercurrent illness, medication), exposures (foods, drinks consumed), outcomes (symptoms) and plausible other exposures which characteristically may be associated with illness (foreign travel, consumption of poultry, etc.) and clinical details about the illness.

33. They are all *measures of central tendency* which assess the location of the middle of the distribution. The *(arithmetic) mean* is what is generally referred to as the average. It is the sum of all scores divided by the total number of scores. For *normal* distributions, the mean is the better measure of central tendency as it does not fluctuate with the sample. The *median* is the central observation of a test, so half the values are above the median and half below it. The *mode* is the most frequently occurring score in a distribution. It should not be used on its own as it fluctuates with the sample and many distributions have more than one mode. The mean, median and mode are identical for symmetric distributions. On the whole, the mean will be higher than the median for *positively skewed* distributions and less than the median for *negatively skewed* distributions.

34. It provides an efficient and systematic way of reviewing vast amounts of medical literature and translating it into good patient care, and a robust way of managing a disease and enhancing the clinical outcome. Furthermore, it serves as a means of modifying current disease-management practices so as to improve the process and can provide a coordinated plan for the management of a disease by the multi-disciplinary team. It also identifies gaps in the current state of knowledge and highlights areas requiring more investigation and allows one to improve the quality and efficiency of disease-management procedures. The common pitfalls encountered in practising evidence-based medicine (EBM) are that a significant proportion of clinicians lack formal training and time and are not able to thoroughly evaluate some research studies. It is easier to read from a textbook even though it may be out of date. There is also a lack of EBM guidelines at the point of practice, e.g. the wards.

35.
   (a) Improve the quality of care and hence patient outcomes.
   (b) The process should be led by clinicians directly involved in patient care.
   (c) It is a multi-disciplinary team activity.
   (d) It examines clinical issues such as diagnosis, treatment and patient care.
   (e) It involves setting standards and measuring against them.
   (f) Finally, an audit involves changing our everyday practice to remedy any deficiencies.

References

Mechanic D 1978 Medical Sociology. New York: The Free Press, pp. 268–287

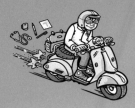

Index

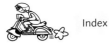

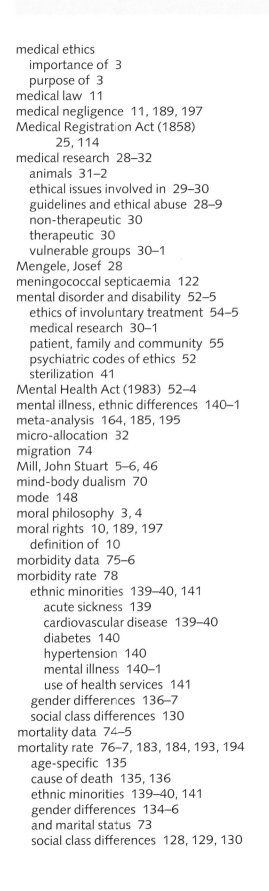

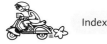

Index